Reflections on Sharing Clinical Trial Data

Challenges and a Way Forward

PROCEEDINGS OF A WORKSHOP

Theresa Wizemann, Eeshan Khandekar, Jennifer Hinners, and Carolyn Shore, *Rapporteurs*

Forum on Drug Discovery, Development, and Translation
Forum on Neuroscience and Nervous System Disorders
National Cancer Policy Forum
Roundtable on Genomics and Precision Health

Board on Health Sciences Policy
Board on Health Care Services

Health and Medicine Division

The National Academies of
SCIENCES · ENGINEERING · MEDICINE

THE NATIONAL ACADEMIES PRESS
Washington, DC
www.nap.edu

THE NATIONAL ACADEMIES PRESS 500 Fifth Street, NW Washington, DC 20001

This activity was supported by contracts between the National Academy of Sciences and AbbVie Inc.; Amgen Inc. (Contract No. GHCCOPS-CSARF-175837); Association of American Medical Colleges; AstraZeneca; Burroughs Wellcome Fund (Contract No. 1020264); Critical Path Institute; Eli Lilly and Company (Contract No. 4900709231); FasterCures, Milken Institute; Foundation for the National Institutes of Health; Friends of Cancer Research; GlaxoSmithKline (Contract No. OTH-PPL-30507 and Contract No. OTH-PPL-32245); Johnson & Johnson; Merck & Co., Inc. (Contract No. MRLCPO-18-2641 and Contract No. MRLCPO-19-106723); National Institutes of Health (Contract No. HHSN263201800029I; Task Order No. HHSN26300007): National Cancer Institute, National Center for Advancing Translational Sciences, National Institute of Allergy and Infectious Diseases, National Institute of Mental Health, National Institute of Neurological Disorders and Stroke, Office of Extramural Research, Office of Science Policy; *New England Journal of Medicine*; Takeda Pharmaceuticals (Contract No. 53108); U.S. Food and Drug Administration (Grant No. 5R13FD005496-04 and Grant No. 5R13FD005496-05); and Wellcome Trust. Any opinions, findings, conclusions, or recommendations expressed in this publication do not necessarily reflect the views of any organization or agency that provided support for the project.

International Standard Book Number-13: 978-0-309-67915-2
International Standard Book Number-10: 0-309-67915-X
Digital Object Identifier: https://doi.org/10.17226/25838

Additional copies of this publication are available from the National Academies Press, 500 Fifth Street, NW, Keck 360, Washington, DC 20001; (800) 624-6242 or (202) 334-3313; http://www.nap.edu.

Printed in the United States of America

Suggested citation: National Academies of Sciences, Engineering, and Medicine. 2020. *Reflections on sharing clinical trial data: Challenges and a way forward: Proceedings of a workshop*. Washington, DC: The National Academies Press. https://doi.org/10.17226/25838.

The National Academies of

SCIENCES • ENGINEERING • MEDICINE

The **National Academy of Sciences** was established in 1863 by an Act of Congress, signed by President Lincoln, as a private, nongovernmental institution to advise the nation on issues related to science and technology. Members are elected by their peers for outstanding contributions to research. Dr. Marcia McNutt is president.

The **National Academy of Engineering** was established in 1964 under the charter of the National Academy of Sciences to bring the practices of engineering to advising the nation. Members are elected by their peers for extraordinary contributions to engineering. Dr. John L. Anderson is president.

The **National Academy of Medicine** (formerly the Institute of Medicine) was established in 1970 under the charter of the National Academy of Sciences to advise the nation on medical and health issues. Members are elected by their peers for distinguished contributions to medicine and health. Dr. Victor J. Dzau is president.

The three Academies work together as the **National Academies of Sciences, Engineering, and Medicine** to provide independent, objective analysis and advice to the nation and conduct other activities to solve complex problems and inform public policy decisions. The National Academies also encourage education and research, recognize outstanding contributions to knowledge, and increase public understanding in matters of science, engineering, and medicine.

Learn more about the National Academies of Sciences, Engineering, and Medicine at **www.nationalacademies.org**.

The National Academies of
SCIENCES · ENGINEERING · MEDICINE

PLANNING COMMITTEE ON SHARING CLINICAL TRIAL DATA: CHALLENGES AND A WAY FORWARD[1]

JEFFREY M. DRAZEN (*Co-Chair*), *New England Journal of Medicine*
JOANNE WALDSTREICHER (*Co-Chair*), Johnson & Johnson
MONICA BERTAGNOLLI, Harvard Medical School; Dana-Farber Cancer Institute and Brigham and Women's Hospital
TIMOTHY COETZEE, National Multiple Sclerosis Society
PATRICK CULLINAN, bluebird bio
SONALI KOCHHAR, Global Healthcare Consulting; University of Washington; Erasmus MC, University Medical Center
BERNARD LO, The Greenwall Foundation
DEVEN McGRAW, Ciitizen Corporation
DINA PALTOO, National Library of Medicine, National Institutes of Health
LIZ ROBERTS, UCB Biosciences, Inc.
FRANK ROCKHOLD, Duke University Medical Center
SHARON TERRY, Genetic Alliance
DEBORAH ZARIN, Multi-Regional Clinical Trials Center of Brigham and Women's Hospital and Harvard

Health and Medicine Division Staff

CAROLYN SHORE, Director, Forum on Drug Discovery, Development, and Translation
JENNIFER HINNERS, Program Officer
EESHAN KHANDEKAR, Associate Program Officer
MELVIN JOPPY, Senior Program Assistant
ANDREW M. POPE, Senior Director, Board on Health Sciences Policy

Consultant

THERESA WIZEMANN, Science Writer

[1] The National Academies of Sciences, Engineering, and Medicine's planning committees are solely responsible for organizing the workshop, identifying topics, and choosing speakers. The responsibility for the published Proceedings of a Workshop rests with the workshop rapporteurs and the institution.

FORUM ON DRUG DISCOVERY, DEVELOPMENT, AND TRANSLATION[1]

[1] The National Academies of Sciences, Engineering, and Medicine's forums and roundtables do not issue, review, or approve individual documents. The responsibility for the published Proceedings of a Workshop rests with the workshop rapporteurs and the institution.

Forum Staff

CAROLYN SHORE, Forum Director
JENNIFER HINNERS, Program Officer
AMANDA WAGNER GEE, Program Officer
EESHAN KHANDEKAR, Associate Program Officer
SYLVIA NCHA, Associate Program Officer
MELVIN JOPPY, Senior Program Assistant
ANDREW M. POPE, Senior Director, Board on Health Sciences Policy

JOSEPH P. MENETSKI, Foundation for the National Institutes of Health
CAROLINE MONTOJO, The Kavli Foundation
STEVEN PAUL, Voyager Therapeutics
EMILIANGELO RATTI, Takeda Pharmaceuticals International
TODD SHERER, The Michael J. Fox Foundation for Parkinson's Research
DAVID SHURTLEFF, National Center for Complementary and Integrative Health
SANTA TUMMINIA, National Eye Institute
NORA VOLKOW, National Institute on Drug Abuse
ANDREW WELCHMAN, Wellcome Trust
DOUG WILLIAMSON, Lundbeck
STEVIN ZORN, MindImmune Therapeutics, Inc.

Forum Staff

CLARE STROUD, Forum Director
SHEENA M. POSEY NORRIS, Program Officer
PHOENIX WILSON, Senior Program Assistant
ANDREW M. POPE, Senior Director, Board on Health Sciences Policy

NATIONAL CANCER POLICY FORUM

EDWARD J. BENZ, JR. (*Chair*), Dana-Farber Cancer Institute and Harvard Medical School
GARNET L. ANDERSON, Fred Hutchinson Cancer Research Center and University of Washington
KENNETH ANDERSON, American Cancer Society and Jerome Lipper Multiple Myeloma Center
KAREN BASEN-ENGQUIST, The University of Texas MD Anderson Cancer Center
LINDA BOHANNON, Cancer Support Community
CHRIS BOSHOFF, Pfizer Inc.
CATHY J. BRADLEY, Colorado School of Public Health and University of Colorado Cancer Center
OTIS W. BRAWLEY, Johns Hopkins University
CYNTHIA BROGDON, Bristol-Myers Squibb Company
ROBERT W. CARLSON, National Comprehensive Cancer Network
GWEN DARIEN, National Patient Advocate Foundation
NANCY E. DAVIDSON, Seattle Cancer Care Alliance; Fred Hutchinson Cancer Research Center; and University of Washington
GEORGE D. DEMETRI, Harvard Medical School; Dana-Farber Cancer Institute; and Dana-Farber/Harvard Cancer Center
JAMES H. DOROSHOW, National Cancer Institute
NICOLE F. DOWLING, Centers for Disease Control and Prevention
SCOT W. EBBINGHAUS, Merck Research Laboratories
KOJO S. J. ELENITOBA-JOHNSON, University of Pennsylvania
STANTON L. GERSON, Case Western Reserve University and University Hospitals Seidman Cancer Center
LORI HOFFMAN HÖGG, U.S. Department of Veterans Affairs
HEDVIG HRICAK, Memorial Sloan Kettering Cancer Center
ERIN HUFMAN, Novartis Oncology
ROY A. JENSEN, Association of American Cancer Institutes; The University of Kansas Cancer Center; and Kansas Masonic Cancer Research Institute
LISA KENNEDY SHELDON, Oncology Nursing Society
SAMIR N. KHLEIF, Georgetown University Medical Center
MICHELLE M. LE BEAU, University of Chicago Medicine Comprehensive Cancer Center
MIA LEVY, Rush University Cancer Center and Rush System for Health
J. LEONARD LICHTENFELD, American Cancer Society
NEAL J. MEROPOL, Flatiron Health
MARTIN J. MURPHY, CEO Roundtable on Cancer

RANDALL A. OYER, Penn Medicine Lancaster General Health
RICHARD L. SCHILSKY, American Society of Clinical Oncology
JULIE SCHNEIDER, U.S. Food and Drug Administration
DEBORAH SCHRAG, Harvard Medical School and Dana-Farber Cancer Institute
LAWRENCE N. SHULMAN, University of Pennsylvania
DAN THEODORESCU, Cedars-Sinai Medical Center
GEORGE J. WEINER, The University of Iowa
ROBERT A. WINN, Virginia Commonwealth University Massey Cancer Center

Forum Staff

ERIN BALOGH, Senior Program Officer
EMILY ZEVON, Associate Program Officer
CYNDI TRANG, Research Associate
KATE HAWTHORNE, Senior Program Assistant
ANNALEE GONZALES, Administrative Assistant
ADEGBOYEGA AKINSIKU, Mirzayan Fellow
SHARYL NASS, Director, National Cancer Policy Forum, and Senior Director, Board on Health Care Services

ROUNDTABLE ON GENOMICS AND PRECISION HEALTH

RYAN TAFT, Illumina
JACQUELYN TAYLOR, New York University
SHARON TERRY, Genetic Alliance
JOYCE TUNG, 23andMe
JAMESON VOSS, Air Force Medical Support Agency
MICHAEL WATSON, American College of Medical Genetics and Genomics
KAREN WECK, College of American Pathologists
CATHERINE WICKLUND, National Society of Genetic Counselors
HUNTINGTON F. WILLARD, Geisinger National Precision Health
JANET WILLIAMS, American Academy of Nursing
SARAH WORDSWORTH, University of Oxford
ALICIA ZHOU, Color Genomics

Roundtable Staff

SARAH BEACHY, Senior Program Officer and Roundtable Director
SIOBHAN ADDIE, Program Officer
MEREDITH HACKMANN, Associate Program Officer
MICHAEL BERRIOS, Senior Program Assistant
ANDREW M. POPE, Senior Director, Board on Health Sciences Policy

Reviewers

This Proceedings of a Workshop was reviewed in draft form by individuals chosen for their diverse perspectives and technical expertise. The purpose of this independent review is to provide candid and critical comments that will assist the National Academies of Sciences, Engineering, and Medicine in making each published proceedings as sound as possible and to ensure that it meets the institutional standards for quality, objectivity, evidence, and responsiveness to the charge. The review comments and draft manuscript remain confidential to protect the integrity of the process.

We thank the following individuals for their review of this proceedings:

TIMOTHY COETZEE, National Multiple Sclerosis Society
ALEXA T. McCRAY, Harvard Medical School
JOHN ORLOFF, Alexion

Although the reviewers listed above provided many constructive comments and suggestions, they were not asked to endorse the content of the proceedings nor did they see the final draft before its release. The review of this proceedings was overseen by **DANIEL MASYS,** University of Washington. He was responsible for making certain that an independent examination of this proceedings was carried out in accordance with standards of the National Academies and that all review comments were carefully considered. Responsibility for the final content rests entirely with the rapporteurs and the National Academies.

Acknowledgments

Sponsorship from the Wellcome Trust helped make this workshop possible. Support from the sponsors of the National Academies of Sciences, Engineering, and Medicine's Forum on Drug Discovery, Development, and Translation; Forum on Neuroscience and Nervous System Disorders; National Cancer Policy Forum; and Roundtable on Genomics and Precision Health is crucial to support this and other work of the National Academies.

The National Academies staff wish to express their gratitude to the speakers whose presentations helped inform workshop discussions on the state of clinical trial data sharing; to the members of the planning committee for their work in developing the workshop agenda and shaping the discussions; and to the many other National Academies staff without whom this workshop and the accounting thereof would not have been possible: Jeanay Butler, Robert Day, Sadaf Faraz, Greta Gorman, Anna Isabel Camilo Javier, Bardia Massoudkhan, Bettina Seliber, Lauren Shern, Victor Stewart, and Taryn Young.

Contents

Boxes and Figures

BOXES

FIGURES

Acronyms and Abbreviations

ACCENT	Adjuvant Colon Cancer End Points
ADaM	CDISC Analysis Data Model
ALS	amyotrophic lateral sclerosis
APC	Adenoma Prevention with Celecoxib
APPROVe	Adenomatous Polyp Prevention on Vioxx Trial
BMS	Bristol-Myers Squibb
BRIDG	Biomedical Research Integrated Domain Group
CARE	Collective benefit, Authority to control, Responsibility, and Ethics
CDISC	Clinical Data Interchange Standards Consortium
CSDR	ClinicalStudyDataRequest.com
CTSU	Clinical Trial Services Unit and Epidemiological Studies Unit
CTT	Cholesterol Treatment Trialists' Collaboration
dbGaP	database of Genotypes and Phenotypes (National Center for Biotechnology Information)
DCRI	Duke Clinical Research Institute
DSA	data sharing agreement (used interchangeably with DUA)
DSMB	Data and Safety Monitoring Board
DUA	data use agreement (used interchangeably with DSA)
EHR	electronic health record

FAIR	findable, accessible, interoperable, and reusable
FDA	U.S. Food and Drug Administration
FHIR	Fast Healthcare Interoperability Resources
ICMJE	International Committee of Medical Journal Editors
ICTRP	International Clinical Trials Registry Platform (WHO)
IDDO	Infectious Diseases Data Observatory
IOM	Institute of Medicine
IPD	individual participant data or individual patient data
IRB	institutional review board
IRP	independent review panel
ITT	intention to treat
LDL	low-density lipoprotein
MIT	Massachusetts Institute of Technology
MRC	Medical Research Council (United Kingdom)
NCI	National Cancer Institute
NCORP	NCI Community Oncology Research Program
NCTN	National Clinical Trials Network (NCI)
NHLBI	National Heart, Lung, and Blood Institute (NIH)
NIH	National Institutes of Health
NMA	network meta-analysis
PEER	Platform for Engaging Everyone Responsibly
SDMC	Statistics and Data Management Center
SDTM	CDISC Study Data Tabulation Model
SOAR	Supporting Open Access for Researchers
SPRINT	Systolic Blood Pressure Intervention Trial
TRS	Trial Reporting System
TSC	Trial Steering Committee
UCL	University College London
WHO	World Health Organization
WWARN	WorldWide Antimalarial Resistance Network
YODA	Yale University Open Data Access Project

1

Introduction[1]

On November 18 and 19, 2019, the National Academies of Sciences, Engineering, and Medicine (the National Academies) hosted a public workshop in Washington, DC, titled Sharing Clinical Trial Data: Challenges and a Way Forward. The workshop followed the release of the 2015 Institute of Medicine (IOM) consensus study report *Sharing Clinical Trial Data: Maximizing Benefits, Minimizing Risk*, and was designed to examine the current state of clinical trial data sharing and reuse and to consider ways in which policy, technology, incentives, and governance could be leveraged to further encourage and enhance data sharing. The workshop planning committee responded to a Statement of Task (see Box 1-1) to develop the workshop agenda and identify speakers to invite.[2] The workshop was sponsored and convened jointly by the Forum on Drug Discovery, Development, and Translation; the Forum on Neuroscience and Nervous System Disorders; the National Cancer Policy Forum; and the Roundtable on Genomics and Precision Health, with additional support from the Wellcome Trust.

---

[1] This workshop was organized by an independent planning committee whose role was limited to identification of topics and speakers. This Proceedings of a Workshop was prepared by the rapporteurs as a factual summary of the presentations and discussion that took place at the workshop. Statements, recommendations, and opinions expressed are those of individual presenters and participants and are not endorsed or verified by the National Academies of Sciences, Engineering, and Medicine, and they should not be construed as reflecting any group consensus.

[2] The workshop agenda can be found in Appendix B. Archived webcast videos and speakers' presentations are available on the National Academies website. See http://nationalacademies.org/hmd/Activities/Research/DrugForum/2019-Nov-18.aspx (accessed February 10, 2020).

BOX 1-1
Workshop Statement of Task

An ad hoc planning committee under the auspices of the National Academies of Sciences, Engineering, and Medicine will plan and conduct a 2-day public workshop to discuss advances, challenges, and opportunities in clinical trial data-sharing efforts since the release of the 2015 Institute of Medicine report *Sharing Clinical Trial Data: Maximizing Benefits, Minimizing Risk*. This workshop is co-sponsored by the Wellcome Trust.

The public workshop will feature invited presentations and discussions to:

- Consider the value and the potential risks and costs of sharing clinical trial data for key stakeholders, including clinical trialists, sponsors, primary and secondary researchers,[a] and patients;
- Review the current landscape of clinical trial data sharing and reuse across public and private sectors (e.g., policies, platforms, collaborations, data-sharing culture, published research output);
- Examine use cases and trends from across public and private sectors when it comes to success, failure, lessons learned, and value;
- Consider the perspectives and expectations of primary and secondary researchers, clinical trial participants, patient organizations, research sponsors (pharmaceutical companies and nonprofit organizations), journals, institutions, and federal agencies; and
- Discuss next-step opportunities for stakeholders to better harmonize incentives, policies, data standards, and governance to encourage the sharing and reuse of clinical trial data.

The planning committee will organize the workshop, develop the agenda, select and invite speakers and discussants, and moderate or identify moderators for the discussions. Proceedings of the presentations and discussions at the workshop will be prepared by a designated rapporteur in accordance with institutional guidelines.

[a] In this summary "primary researcher" is used interchangeably with "data generator," and "secondary researcher" is used interchangeably with "data user."

This workshop also builds on a body of related activities, including the IOM workshop summaries *Envisioning a Transformed Clinical Trials Enterprise in the United States: Establishing an Agenda for 2020* (IOM, 2012a) and *Sharing Clinical Research Data* (IOM, 2013) and other National Academies publications discussing the sharing and reuse of clinical trial data.[3]

[3] A collection of National Academies publications on clinical trial data sharing is available at https://www.nap.edu/collection/90/clinical-trial-data-sharing (accessed March 2, 2020).

REVISITING THE 2015 INSTITUTE OF MEDICINE CONSENSUS STUDY REPORT *SHARING CLINICAL TRIAL DATA: MAXIMIZING BENEFITS, MINIMIZING RISK*

Joanne Waldstreicher, chief medical officer at Johnson & Johnson and co-chair of the workshop, highlighted that the 2015 study outlined guiding principles for the sharing of individual participant data (IPD) from clinical trials and issued recommendations regarding the roles and responsibilities of key stakeholders, the timeframe in which data should be shared, and considerations for access to and governance of shared clinical trial data (IOM, 2015). The 2015 IOM study did not address the sharing of real-world data, such as the information contained in patient electronic health records or administrative data from health insurance claims, she added. Jeffrey M. Drazen, *New England Journal of Medicine* group editor and co-chair of the workshop, clarified that the 2015 study focused on data from clinical trials for two reasons: (1) data obtained from clinical trials are of high quality, and (2) individuals put themselves at risk and relinquish control of aspects of their clinical care when they participate in a clinical study. He emphasized the difficulty of enrolling participants who satisfy inclusion criteria for the study, and who are available and willing to participate.

Bernard Lo, president and chief executive officer of The Greenwall Foundation and chair of the 2015 IOM study, provided a brief overview of the report's recommendations (see Box 1-2 for the full text). The first recommendation called for establishing a culture of data sharing, which could include, Lo summarized, considering data sharing for academic promotion and requiring data-sharing provisions in research grant proposals. The second recommendation addressed the types of clinical trial data to be shared and the timeline for sharing. The third recommendation provided guidance on operational strategies to facilitate clinical trial data sharing, such as the needs for independent review panels to assess requests for access to data and transparency surrounding the availability and accessibility of clinical trial data. The fourth recommendation called for an ongoing, multi-stakeholder process to address the structural and logistical elements of data sharing.

PROGRESS MADE IN CLINICAL TRIAL DATA SHARING SINCE THE 2015 INSTITUTE OF MEDICINE CONSENSUS STUDY REPORT

To reflect on progress made in clinical trial data sharing since the release of the 2015 IOM consensus study report *Sharing Clinical Trial Data: Maximizing Benefits, Minimizing Risk,* Drazen said that data collected during randomized controlled clinical trials were originally considered to

BOX 1-2
Recommendations from the 2015 Institute of Medicine Consensus Study Report *Sharing Clinical Trial Data: Maximizing Benefits, Minimizing Risk*

- "RECOMMENDATION 1: Stakeholders in clinical trials should foster a culture in which data sharing is the expected norm, and should commit to responsible strategies aimed at maximizing the benefits, minimizing the risks, and overcoming the challenges of sharing clinical trial data for all parties.
- RECOMMENDATION 2: Sponsors and investigators should share the various types of clinical trial data no later than the times specified in this report (e.g., the full analyzable dataset with metadata no later than 18 months after study completion—with specified exceptions for trials intended to support a regulatory application—and the analytic dataset supporting publication results no later than 6 months after publication).
- RECOMMENDATION 3: Holders of clinical trial data should mitigate the risks and enhance the benefits of sharing sensitive clinical trial data by implementing operational strategies that include employing data use agreements, designating an independent review panel, including members of the lay public in governance, and making access to clinical trial data transparent.
- RECOMMENDATION 4: The sponsors of this study should take the lead, together with or via a trusted impartial organization(s), to convene a multistakeholder body with global reach and broad representation to address, in an ongoing process, the key infrastructure, technological, sustainability, and workforce challenges associated with the sharing of clinical trial data."

SOURCE: IOM, 2015, p. xiv.

be the property of those who conducted the study. As data science and technology have evolved to better enable researchers to analyze large volumes of data, discussions regarding data ownership and the need for data sharing have continued to advance. Today, Drazen said, the focus is on finding ways to share clinical trial data for the benefit of key stakeholder groups: the clinical trial participants who put themselves at risk, the skilled clinical trialists who gather the high-quality data, and the data scientists who mine and analyze the data for new insights. The task, he said, is to define the value of shared data and align incentives for sharing for the benefit of human health.

"Spirited disagreement" persists among data generators and data users regarding how, when, and whether to share clinical trial data, Lo said. Data generators (i.e., clinical trialists), for example, expend great effort in planning and executing a trial and might believe that they are due long-term usage rights. On the other hand, Lo continued, data users are eager to use clinical trial data for secondary analyses to answer current questions. The challenge, he emphasized, is to arrive at data-sharing terms that recognize both perspectives and meet the ultimate goal of providing benefit to patients.

Lo suggested that debates about data sharing can be evidence driven and that metrics are needed for measuring benefits and values. An objective of data sharing is to generate and operationalize important new knowledge, he added. However, it is unclear whether secondary analyses of clinical trial data do, in fact, generate new knowledge. Therefore, metrics that reflect whether sharing of clinical trial data leads to improved health and clinical outcomes could be considered. But there is still a question as to whether all clinical trials should have equal priority for data sharing, he continued. Some trials might provide greater value or benefit from data sharing than others. For example, sharing data from a large-scale, multi-center, pivotal clinical trial that was designed to impact clinical practice could be of high value. There are also opportunity costs that should be recognized and quantified, Lo concluded (e.g., external parties may beat investigators to conducting planned secondary analyses as a result of trial data being simultaneously released with publication, and may be a disincentive in clinical research).

Sharing Individual Participant Data

Deborah Zarin, director of the Program for Advancement of the Clinical Trial Enterprise at Brigham and Women's Hospital and Harvard, illustrated the current clinical Trial Reporting System (TRS) conceptually as a pyramid (see Figure 1-1). The foundation of a TRS is the prospective registration of trials in a public database (e.g., ClinicalTrials.gov) that provides a searchable record of ongoing and completed clinical trials. Registry entries include key protocol details, which enable users to search for trials in a research area of interest and to track the progress of a study. The next level includes summary results reporting, in which a minimum set of aggregate data from trials is reported in a structured and searchable format in a trial registry, with links to peer-reviewed journal articles. At the top of the pyramid is the sharing of IPD.

Zarin noted the need for clarity regarding what is meant by "data" and "sharing" when discussing IPD sharing. The value of IPD varies as it is transformed from raw data (e.g., case report forms) to aggregated and coded datasets. The type, quality, and usability of the metadata (e.g., definition of variables) are also important. Sharing is generally considered to be the process of making the data available for independent use by another research team, Zarin said. Zarin continued that opinions vary, however, regarding the extent to which the original research team

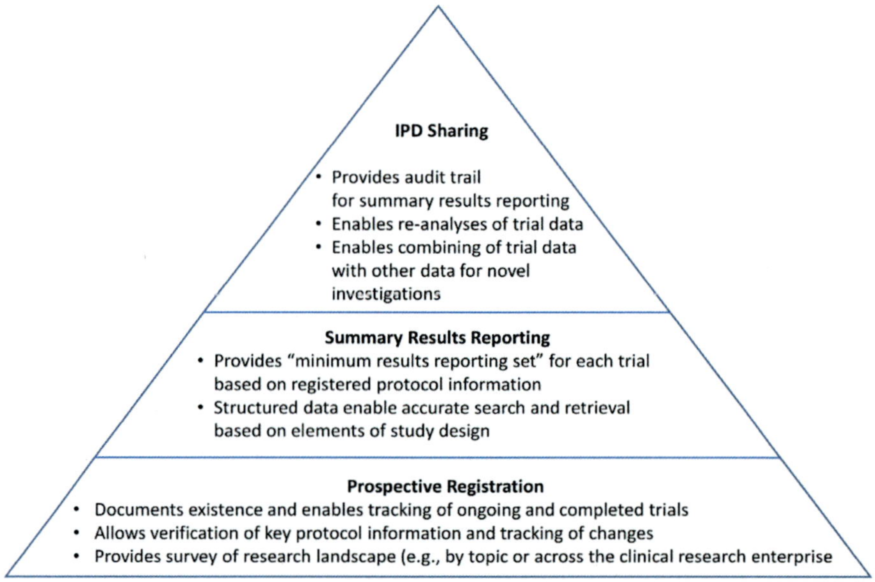

FIGURE 1-1 Functions of the Trial Reporting System.
NOTE: IPD = individual participant data.
SOURCES: As presented by Deborah Zarin, November 18, 2019; Zarin and Tse, 2016.

that collected the data should remain involved. The value of data can be impacted by whether data sharing is active (i.e., proactively made available) or latent (i.e., whether the data generator expects that others will ever look at their data). It is human nature, she said, to behave differently when someone might be observing. For example, Zarin explained, the pharmaceutical industry expects that all clinical data it generates will be reviewed by regulatory authorities, and data are collected, documented, and analyzed accordingly. In contrast, researchers in academia generally do not expect that level of external review of their data. Given that all data might not be of equal priority for sharing, Zarin suggested it may be useful to think about what balance of sharing (active versus latent) would be appropriate. One question she posed for consideration is whether making all trials at risk for audit would enhance value.

To put IPD sharing in the TRS in context, Zarin shared recent statistics from the ClinicalTrials.gov database. Most clinical trials appear to be registered, she said, although about one-third of these trials were registered late (more than 3 months after the start of the trial). Zarin stated that ideally, every trial that is registered should have summary results reported on ClinicalTrials.gov. However, not all registered trials are conducted or completed, so the number of registered trials and the number of summary results reported are not expected to be equal, she explained. Currently, an estimate of only about 50 percent of trials report summary results (directly in the registry or via peer-reviewed publication). Reporting varies by sector and is more common for trials subject to regulation. Few trials registered in ClinicalTrials.gov have links to IPD, Zarin said. For example, out of 4,700 clinical trials completed in 2016 (with at least one U.S. site), only 5 have links to IPD; and only 2 out of about 2,000 drug efficacy studies (Phase 2 and beyond) have links to IPD. In fact, only 653 studies had links to IPD out of 155,000 completed studies in ClinicalTrials.gov, Zarin noted. The International Committee of Medical Journal Editors (ICMJE) instituted a policy that, starting in 2019, all trials must provide a data-sharing plan registering to be considered for publication in an ICMJE journal.[4] Looking at the 7,309 clinical trials launched in 2019 (registered in ClinicalTrials.gov with a site in the United States), Zarin found that 1,120 (15 percent) have declared the intention to share IPD (3,749 declared they would not share IPD, and 2,440 were undecided or did not respond).

In summary, Zarin said that about half of the trials registered in ClinicalTrials.gov report summary results, and a very small fraction report IPD. She emphasized that, although IPD sharing is important, trial registration and summary results reporting form the foundation of the evidence base. In addition, failure to share IPD via a searchable system that is linked to trial registration and summary results can lead to reporting bias. She prompted workshop participants to consider what the goals of IPD sharing should be. Is a low burden of posting and using IPD desirable? Should there be a target percentage of trials with IPD available, and if so, what would the target be? Should all trials be at risk of audit? Is the ultimate goal of sharing IPD to facilitate high-impact discoveries? Finally, what indicators might suggest that a change of strategy for sharing of IPD is warranted?

ORGANIZATION OF THE WORKSHOP AND PROCEEDINGS

This Proceedings of a Workshop summarizes the presentations and discussions that took place at the workshop. Following the introductory remarks (Chapter 1), the first three workshop panels considered the current landscape for clinical trial data sharing and reuse. Panelists shared their perspectives on current data-sharing policies in practice (Chapter 2), described case examples of data-sharing platforms (Chapter 3), and discussed balancing the value and benefits of sharing data with the risks

[4] See http://www.icmje.org/recommendations/browse/publishing-and-editorial-issues/clinical-trial-registration.html#two (accessed February 10, 2020).

and costs (Chapter 4). The next three panels considered some of the key challenges to clinical trial data sharing and reuse. Panelists discussed data interoperability and platform usability (Chapter 5) and infrastructure sustainability (Chapter 6) and examined challenges and disincentives for sharing in the context of statistical replication (Chapter 7). The final two panels of the workshop focused on moving data sharing forward. Panelists explored opportunities for overcoming the technical and sustainability challenges discussed (Chapter 8) and considered steps to incentivize and promote data sharing and reuse (Chapter 9).

2

Perspectives on Current Data-Sharing Policies in Practice

Highlights of Key Points Made by Individual Speakers

- Sharing data brings new perspectives and ideas to the analyses and can lead to new insights that serve the public good. Not sharing data is wasteful and may result in missed opportunities to learn. (Krumholz)
- Researchers benefit from data that are shared by others, but may be hesitant to share their own data. This is due, in part, to the academic culture, which does not recognize, reward, or incentivize data sharing or team science. (Krumholz)
- Data sharing facilitates accountability to trial participants, allowing them to see how their time and data can help move clinical science forward. (Jorgenson)
- Trial participants do not necessarily perceive any disadvantage to widely sharing their clinical trial data and generally consider that data sharing is beneficial. (Taylor)
- Other than being asked to consent to sharing of their data, trial participants generally receive little or no information about what will be done with the data that are generated from a given study. (Taylor)
- Volumes of data are now available for request and analysis, but incentives and approaches that can enhance data sharing and reuse are needed. (Kochhar)

- Independent review panels can help ensure that data-sharing platforms provide data access to secondary users in a consistent, transparent, trusted, and controlled manner. (Kochhar)
- Metrics are needed to better understand whether information about clinical trial participation is useful and understandable to the public; to assess and track the scientific value of clinical trial data; and to understand if and how data are being shared and/or reused. (Jorgenson)

The first workshop panel considered the current landscape for clinical trial data sharing and reuse, and provided stakeholder perspectives on current data-sharing policies in practice. Harlan Krumholz, Harold H. Hines Jr. Professor of Medicine at the Yale School of Medicine, discussed the challenges that researchers face as both data generators and users of data generated by others. Moses Taylor, Jr., spoke from his personal experience as a clinical trial participant. Sonali Kochhar, medical director of Global Healthcare Consulting, discussed facilitating data sharing from her perspective as a member of an independent review panel. Lyric Jorgenson, deputy director in the Office of Science Policy at the National Institutes of Health (NIH), discussed data-sharing policies from the perspective of a funder. The panel discussion was moderated by Bernard Lo.

RESEARCHER PERSPECTIVE

Harlan Krumholz, Harold H. Hines Jr. Professor of Medicine, Yale School of Medicine

Sharing his perspective as both a data generator and a user of data generated by others, Krumholz said that unshared data are wasteful, result in missed opportunities to learn, and do not serve the public good. Researchers are faced with a host of "incentives to sequester data" for themselves, he said. He acknowledged the progress that has been made in facilitating transparent sharing of clinical trial data, such as the Yale University Open Data Access Project,[1] and expressed optimism about the opportunities to continue to enhance data sharing.

As a researcher, Krumholz said he has benefited from having access to data generated by others. As an example, he described revisiting data from the mid-1990s clinical trial of digoxin for the management of heart failure. The National Heart, Lung, and Blood Institute (NHLBI), which sponsored

[1] See https://yoda.yale.edu (accessed March 2, 2020). Discussed further by Ross in Chapter 3.

the study, had made the data available for analysis, but for years this resource had not been leveraged. Krumholz and colleagues published two secondary analyses, which he said sparked interest from the original NHLBI investigators and other investigators in analyzing the dataset for new insights.[2] These subsequent analyses "were complementary and synergistic and served the public good," he said.

Krumholz also spoke from the perspective of a data generator, describing the "emotional distress" of having to share the resulting data from a challenging, multi-site clinical trial he conducted. Researchers often have a social/emotional perspective (incorrectly, he added) that the data they generate are their own, which can impede progress on data sharing. This can occur, he added, despite their acknowledgment of the public good of data sharing and even though data would not exist without trial participants and a broad range of others on the clinical trial team.

This tension between benefiting from data shared by others and the hesitancy to share generated data is fed by the culture within academia. Krumholz said that academia does not recognize, reward, or incentivize data sharing or team science when evaluating researchers for promotions and grants. Little recognition is given to those who enable the important work done by others. In addition, little to no funding support is available to facilitate data sharing, and the infrastructure for sharing is lacking. However, great advances, Krumholz emphasized, can only occur through team science, which includes other researchers and trial participants. Furthermore, sharing data brings new perspectives and ideas to the analyses. Moving forward will require attention to the incentives and rewards structures for scientists, as well as the funding and infrastructure needed to readily enable sharing.

Alex Sherman, director of the Center for Innovation and Bioinformatics at Massachusetts General Hospital, suggested that an incentive for sharing could be including the data contributor as a co-author on publications that analyze his or her data. He noted that several consortia are already doing so and include a provision in the data sharing agreement (DSA). Tim Feeney from *The BMJ* noted that many journals require preregistration of clinical trials as a condition of consideration for publication. He asked whether there might be a similar role for journals in promoting the sharing of data. Krumholz agreed with the spirit of acknowledging data contributors with authorship, but raised his own personal concerns that the data contributors might not meet the criteria for authorship as currently outlined by the International Committee of Medical Journal Editors for its member journals. He suggested that journal articles could indicate the provenance of the

---

[2] See https://www.nejm.org/doi/full/10.1056/nejmoa021266 (accessed March 30, 2020) and https://jamanetwork.com/journals/jama/fullarticle/195990 (accessed March 30, 2020).

data and promote the prior work, perhaps in the supplemental information for a publication or by including a link that would facilitate tracing back to and crediting the data originator. Amy Nurnberger of the Massachusetts Institute of Technology called attention to the practice of data citation—a practice that allows authors to include references to data similar to how publications are cited. Data citations can include digital object identifiers and can be tracked in the same way that article citations are tracked. Nurnberger mentioned ORCID IDs,[3] which are intended to serve as unique identifiers for individuals in the research community.

PATIENT PERSPECTIVE

Moses Taylor, Jr., Participant, Systolic Blood Pressure Intervention Trial

Taylor shared his perspective as a clinical trial participant, drawing from his personal experience in the Systolic Blood Pressure Intervention Trial (SPRINT)[4] as well as his interactions with other trial participants during the 2017 Aligning Incentives for Sharing Clinical Trial Data summit.[5]

The Benefits and Risks of Sharing and Not Sharing Trial Data

Other than being asked to consent to sharing of their data, trial participants generally receive little or no information about what will be done with the data generated from a given study, Taylor reported. He said participants need a better understanding of the potential benefits and risks associated with data sharing before giving consent. He suggested that trial participants should be involved in decision making about how their data are shared.

Taylor observed that, in his experience, trial participants do not perceive any disadvantage to widely sharing their clinical trial data and generally believe that data sharing is beneficial. Most people participate in a clinical trial for personal benefit, in the hope that the results of the trial will ultimately impact their own clinical care, he said. For patients with life-threatening illnesses, trial participation can be lifesaving, and partici-

---

[3] ORCID IDs are persistent digital identifiers assigned to individual researchers that can be used to associate them with their research outputs. (ORCID was originally derived from Open Researcher and Contributor IDentifier but is now referred to as an ORCID ID.) See https://orcid.org (accessed March 2, 2020).

[4] Information on SPRINT is available at https://www.sprinttrial.org/public/dspHome.cfm (accessed February 10, 2020) and https://clinicaltrials.gov/ct2/show/NCT01206062 (accessed February 10, 2020).

[5] Information about this summit is available at https://challenge.nejm.org/pages/about (accessed March 2, 2020).

pants and their providers need to know the results of the trial as soon as possible. Trial participants are also motivated by the opportunity to help others through their participation. From a patient perspective, Taylor said, there is a belief that if more people conduct secondary analysis on data, there is a better chance that discoveries will be made that will help trial participants and others with the same or similar conditions. Sharing data widely can provide "checks and balances," Taylor added, and helps to reduce unintended bias in interpretation as well as misuse of the data by the original trialists versus if data were otherwise not shared.

Taylor acknowledged the potential for inappropriate use of shared data but believed this risk was fairly low due to the data governance systems in place in the United States. There is also a risk of reidentification of individual participants; but again, he perceived this to be of low risk due to the privacy protections that are in place. He added that, depending on the subject of the trial, participants might not think it is harmful to be identified.

Data from SPRINT were shared over the course of the study and at the conclusion, Taylor recalled. In addition, the "SPRINT Data Analysis Challenge" invited analysts after the conclusion of the study to use the trial dataset in novel ways to identify new findings.[6] Taylor said his experience with sharing the data from SPRINT was positive.

In conclusion, Taylor advocated for sharing trial data widely, under the governance of experts, as it provides great benefit to both study participants and patients like them. The consent process ensures that participants understand the health risks of enrolling in a clinical trial, but they generally do not understand what will be done with the data that are generated, he said. Based on his experience, Taylor said that data sharing is an important indicator of the benefit a trial might have for patients, and he recommended that potential trial participants should be provided information on data-sharing plans to help their decision on whether to participate. Jeffrey M. Drazen noted that participant data might be used to answer questions in the future that cannot be predicted at the time of enrollment and consent. Taylor responded that he personally would accept risk involved with data sharing and he reiterated the importance of informing potential participants about the secondary uses of their data during the consent process so they can make informed decisions.

[6] See https://challenge.nejm.org/pages/about (accessed March 2, 2020). Discussed further by Drazen in Chapter 4.

INDEPENDENT REVIEW PANEL PERSPECTIVE

Sonali Kochhar, Medical Director, Global Healthcare Consulting

Kochhar discussed clinical trial data sharing from her perspective as a member of the Wellcome Trust's Independent Review Panel (IRP) for the data-sharing platforms, ClinicalStudyDataRequest.com (CSDR) and Vivli.[7] A Wellcome Trust survey of its grantees found that researchers share data for a variety of reasons, including requirements by funders or journals; belief that data sharing is a good research practice; and understanding that data sharing can facilitate collaboration as well as enable external validation and replication of results. The survey also found that researchers are concerned about the potential for misuse or misrepresentation of their shared data, the loss of opportunities to publish those data, and the time and effort required to deposit data (van Den Eynden et al., 2016). A survey by Kratz and Strasser (2015) found that researchers share data primarily through direct contact, such as email.

Data-Sharing Platforms

Kochhar suggested that data-sharing platforms can help researchers share data by providing "a standard, transparent access route, independent of the data generator." Platforms can also help protect trial participants and align with patient consent by anonymizing data and restricting data access. In addition, platforms can facilitate metadata searches, and in some cases provide data storage.

Data-sharing platforms also present the following challenges, Kochhar said:

- The cost recovery model (the cost of running the platform might be paid for by the data contributor, the data requester, and/or a central core grant)
- The costs of maintaining secure analysis environments
- The lack of internationally agreed-upon minimum standards for metadata (further complicated when metadata are not in English)
- The lack of sufficient information about a study to assess whether data are worth requesting for a given research analysis

[7] CSDR and Vivli are discussed further in Chapter 3. Information about Vivli is available at https://vivli.org. Information about the CSDR platform is available at https://www.clinicalstudydatarequest.com (accessed February 10, 2020). The charter for the CSDR IRP is available at https://clinicalstudydatarequest.com/Documents/Independent_Review_Panel_Charter.pdf (accessed February 10, 2020).

- The lack of interoperability among platforms (resulting in the need for researchers to search and make requests of multiple platforms)
- The lack of internationally agreed-upon standards for DSAs
- The different governance structures used by platforms

Two examples of data-sharing platforms are CSDR and Vivli. CSDR, established in 2013, is a searchable database of more than 3,000 studies.[8] Briefly, researchers submit proposals to CSDR to request access to data from studies of interest. Requests are approved through a process that includes an IRP, and approved data users must sign a DSA before being provided access to the data in a secure system. There is no charge to access the data for secondary analyses. Kochhar noted that data requesters must also seek approval from their own institutional review boards or ethics committees as required by their institutions. A similar process is employed by Vivli, which currently houses more than 4,000 studies.

The Role of Independent Review Panels

The Wellcome Trust serves as the secretariat for CSDR and Vivli IRPs. Using an IRP helps to ensure that access to the data in the platforms are provided in a consistent, transparent, trusted, and controlled manner, Kochhar explained. The multi-disciplinary IRP includes a layperson in addition to members who are highly experienced in reviewing proposals and who have expertise in global health, clinical research, statistics, and ethics. The IRP also provides constructive feedback to researchers.

To illustrate the process, Kochhar said that a total of 531 research proposals had been submitted to CSDR through August 2019. Of those, 409 met the initial check criteria, and, of those, 338 were approved by the IRP. Of those that were rejected, 60 percent were revised to address IRP feedback, resubmitted, and ultimately accepted (Kochhar noted that similar proposal approval rates have been observed at Vivli). Georgina Humphreys, clinical data sharing manager from Wellcome Trust, added that some attrition is due to requesters withdrawing their requests or not responding to correspondence from the platform. In some cases, she said, researchers are approved for access but never log in or conduct analysis. Kochhar noted that a study sponsor has the right to veto secondary data use requests due to concerns, such as potential conflict of interest or competitive risk. However, this option has not been exercised by a sponsor thus far.

The requests to CSDR have led to 80 published or forthcoming publications, which Kochhar suggested is a low number relative to the time

[8] See https://www.clinicalstudydatarequest.com/Metrics.aspx (accessed March 2, 2020).

and resources invested in the platform. Drazen noted that there are other potential metrics to consider besides publications. For example, secondary analysis of data can inform future clinical trial design. Kochhar agreed but added that thus far most secondary data users have been interested in conducting novel research, not designing future clinical research.

The average time from proposal submission to data access at CSDR is about 6 months, Kochhar said. The longest segment is review and signing of the DSA, which averages just over 3.5 months. Kochhar emphasized that this time could be reduced if institutions accepted a standard DSA. Other factors that impact the timeline include the researchers' responses to IRP questions and review by the sponsor's publication steering committee. Kochhar listed some of the common reasons for IRP rejection of proposals:

- The Plain English summary of the proposal was too technical and/or there was not a clear benefit to patients described.
- The information about the scientific rationale and/or clinical relevance of the proposed research was insufficient and the research plan and aims were unclear.
- The study design, methodology, and/or analysis plan provided insufficient detail or was incorrect.
- The research team did not have the relevant skills, qualifications, or experience to carry out the proposed plan.
- No publication or dissemination plan was submitted.

In conclusion, Kochhar shared suggestions to enhance data sharing and reuse based on lessons learned from the IRP process (see Box 2-1). Volumes of data are now available to request for analysis, she said, and there is a need to incentivize data sharing and reuse. She suggested that guidance from professional bodies on issues such as consent or common DSAs would help promote data sharing. She also noted the need to decrease the time from proposal to data access and reduce the cost of data sharing and reuse.

FUNDER PERSPECTIVE

Lyric Jorgenson, Deputy Director, Office of Science Policy, National Institutes of Health

NIH has long been committed to promoting data sharing. Jorgenson discussed NIH's approach, as a funder, to incentivizing data sharing. NIH recently released a draft policy for comment that calls for researchers to prospectively design a plan for data management and sharing, taking into consideration what data are necessary for replicating and validating the

BOX 2-1
Independent Review Panel Perspective: Suggestions to Enhance Data Sharing

- Research agendas should be developed to drive the sharing and reuse of data. These agendas should be informed by the whole community and define the main questions that need to be answered, Kochhar said.
- The "data access process should be easily discoverable" and transparent, with metrics available to potential users.
- Funders should support capacity-building efforts in low- and middle-income countries because most data access requests originate from high-income countries.
- The consent process for clinical research participants could include a "provision for reuse ... of anonymized [participant] data beyond the original study."
- "In the absence of specific guidance, institutional ethics committees ... should adopt consistent policies [regarding] ... ethics review for secondary use of anonymized data."
- Common data-sharing agreements should be available for data providers.
- Common data standards should be used to reduce the resources needed for secondary analysis.
- Common metrics should be used across different data-sharing platforms (e.g., numbers and types of requests, approval dates, reasons for rejection, summary data with links to publications).
- Academic funders should encourage grantees to share clinical research data.

SOURCES: Kochhar presentation, November 18, 2019; Kochhar et al., 2019.

findings of the study.[9] Plans should include timelines for sharing, where data will be shared, and anticipated costs of sharing, she said. Although the default should be to share data, she said that NIH recognizes there are circumstances in which sharing might not be appropriate (e.g., where prohibited by state or tribal laws, or where sharing data is not in the best interest of the research participants). The intent is to submit information to the repository that will enable others to replicate and validate the study.

Jorgenson highlighted the three main reasons NIH is investing significantly in sharing data from clinical trials:

[9] Jorgenson referred participants to the Draft Data Management and Sharing Policy that was recently released by NIH for public comment, available at https://osp.od.nih.gov/scientific-sharing/nih-data-management-and-sharing-activities-related-to-public-access-and-open-science (accessed February 10, 2020).

1. **Sharing clinical trial data supports the concept of engaging participants as partners in research.** People are no longer referred to as research "subjects," Jorgenson said. The focus is now on including them in discussions of study design and how their data are used now and in the future. Data sharing provides accountability, allowing trial participants to see how their time and data help to move clinical science forward.
2. **Sharing clinical trial data supports the accountability and transparency of NIH as a public funder of clinical trials.** NIH invests an estimated $3 billion annually in clinical trials,[10] Jorgenson said. As a public agency, NIH must demonstrate that it is a good steward of taxpayer-funded research and that the sharing and reuse of data are important metrics.
3. **Sharing clinical trial data advances science.** Jorgenson emphasized the importance of sharing all data, both positive clinical trial findings that might impact care as well as negative data that can inform future research and avoid waste of time and resources. NIH is focused on enhancing the value of data generated in clinical trials through prospective planning (e.g., data elements to be collected, where data will be shared).

Metrics

Measures of success are needed for data sharing as it relates to participant engagement and public trust in the clinical research enterprise. Metrics are needed to better understand whether information about clinical trials is useful and understandable to the public, Jorgenson said. Other metrics are needed to evaluate whether the public is willing to participate in clinical trials, whether participants understand the purpose of a given trial, and how participants' data may or may not be used.

Metrics are also needed to assess and track the scientific value of the clinical trial data, as well as the ease with which the data can be shared, Jorgenson said. This involves understanding factors related to how sharing is facilitated—including the standards for data collection, the infrastructure for data sharing (e.g., platforms, repositories), and the processes for accessing human data (e.g., consent, appropriate use). Jorgenson noted that the variability in how data are reported is a key challenge in data sharing.

Also discussed was understanding the importance of whether and how data are being shared and/or reused. Jorgenson observed that

[10] See https://www.nih.gov/about-nih/who-we-are/nih-director/statements/nih-reaches-another-milestone-toward-clinical-trial-stewardship-reforms (accessed March 2, 2020).

researchers' concerns about data sharing and use span the spectrum, from being "scooped" (i.e., by sharing their data they are at risk for others publishing their findings before they do) to having their data go unused.

Challenges and Opportunities

One challenge to sharing clinical trial data is meeting the needs of the different stakeholders that NIH serves. Jorgenson pointed out that the level of granularity needed by scientists is different from that needed by the public. She said that ClinicalTrials.gov continuously strives to strike a balance between providing the level of detail needed by researchers, and providing understandable, usable information for members of the public who are seeking to participate in a trial. Another challenge is meeting infrastructure needs, including physical storage capacity as well as technical knowledge to ensure that data are findable and usable. Shared data, including associated metadata, need to be accessible to be used.

One area where NIH is focusing attention is understanding the value of sharing individual participant data. Jorgenson said that a small pilot study done by NIH of several data repositories found that researchers were accessing individual participant data and combining it with other datasets to pursue new lines of inquiry. It was also found that the reuse of shared data contributes to patents, systematic reviews, and guidelines, she said.

In closing, Jorgenson said that, as a funder, NIH is working to implement policies that incentivize a culture of data sharing. For example, as discussed by Krumholz, there might be approaches that could be used to reward those who generate and share data that are of value and that enable the work of other researchers. In response to a question from Rebecca Li, Jorgenson elaborated that potential incentives include finding ways to make data sharing easier by, for example, reducing administrative hurdles, improving infrastructure for sharing, and supporting cost allowances.

3

Data-Sharing Platforms

Highlights of Key Points Made by Individual Speakers

- Data-sharing platforms should be flexible to meet the needs of individual users; data governance models should incorporate input from a variety of stakeholders. (Li)
- A nonprofit organization that manages a data-sharing platform can help enable data sharing, but other stakeholders in the broader research ecosystem (e.g., funders, publishers, academia) hold the major levers to reward investigators for sharing data. (Li)
- Data-sharing platforms have already presented new opportunities for conducting studies, as well as direct collaborations between researchers and original data contributors. (Ross)
- Concerns about potential unintended consequences of data sharing have not materialized (e.g., participant privacy breaches, undermining of original study findings, commercial or litigious use of data). (Ross)
- The supply of data available for sharing is much greater than the demand for it, and there is a need to raise researcher awareness of the rich data resources that are available to them. (Li, Ross)
- The majority of data requesters are from academia (Rockhold, Ross) while much of the clinical trial data sharing thus far has been carried out by industry. (Rockhold)

- To foster open science and data-sharing academia needs to find a way to provide academic credit for researchers who share original data. (Rockhold)
- To conduct a study across multiple clinical trials that are housed in different data-sharing platforms, researchers often must submit multiple separate data requests, conduct parallel analyses in the different platforms, and then attempt to combine the results. (Shaunessy)
- Data-sharing platforms and companies should work together to identify solutions that allow studies to combine data across platforms. (Shaunessy)
- Data use agreement (DUA) negotiations can cause significant delays during the data request process. A single, harmonized master DUA could improve the data user experience by increasing the efficiency of the data request process. (Li, Ross, Shaunessy)

The second panel presented four current examples of data-sharing repositories. Rebecca Li, executive director of Vivli, shared lessons learned from the Vivli platform since its launch in 2018. Joseph Ross, professor of medicine and public health at the Yale School of Medicine, discussed the operations and impact of the Yale University Open Data Access Project. Frank Rockhold, professor of biostatistics and bioinformatics at the Duke Clinical Research Institute (DCRI), described the multicomponent data-sharing process used by the Supporting Open Access for Researchers (SOAR) platform. Scott Shaunessy, co-founder and chair of ClinicalStudyDataRequest.com (CSDR), discussed challenges and solutions associated with launching CSDR, one of the first data-sharing platforms. The panel discussion was moderated by Deborah Zarin.

Additional details about each of the platforms were provided on posters that were available in the meeting room throughout the workshop.[1]

VIVLI

Rebecca Li, Executive Director, Vivli

Vivli is a nonprofit organization focused on clinical research data sharing that provides a convening function for stakeholders in biomedical

[1] The posters presented are available on the workshop webpage, http://nationalacademies.org/hmd/Activities/Research/DrugForum/2019-Nov-18.aspx (accessed February 10, 2020), under the Attachments menu.

research, including industry, academia, nonprofit funders and foundations, government, and patient advocates.[2] Launched in July 2018, Vivli houses a clinical trial data-sharing platform also called Vivli, Li explained.

Since its inception, more than 4,600 clinical trials have been contributed to the Vivli platform by Vivli members.[3] The trials include data from more than 2 million participants from more than 100 countries. Vivli has met strong and sustained enthusiasm, Li said. During the repository's first year, more than 80 data request proposals were submitted, and data from more than 80 trials involving approximately 65,000 participants were accessed. Li added that the platform is anticipated to achieve financial sustainability in the first quarter of 2020. Searches of the repository span a broad range of outcomes, diseases, and products. Zarin asked about the extent to which trials contributed to Vivli link back to their ClinicalTrials.gov registry entry. Li said that some members are starting to carry out such linking, but some have expressed concern about the need to update the entire ClinicalTrials.gov record retrospectively.

The Vivli Model

The 2015 Institute of Medicine (IOM) consensus study report *Sharing Clinical Trial Data: Maximizing Benefits, Minimizing Risk* (IOM, 2015) was used as a blueprint in the development of the Vivli platform, Li said. Vivli strives to uphold the report's general principles, especially "conducting the sharing of trial data in a fair manner." Vivli uses the flowchart for what data to share and when from the 2015 IOM report when training new members,[4] and employs a harmonized data use agreement (DUA). As mentioned by Kochhar (see Chapter 2), the Wellcome Trust is the secretariat for the Vivli independent review panel (IRP), although some Vivli members choose to use their own IRP. In achieving sustainability, Li said that Vivli is a membership-driven model and operates under the principle expressed in the IOM report that those who benefit from data sharing should also be responsible for contributing financially (IOM, 2015). Vivli is also working toward becoming more searchable and interoperable, she said.

[2] Further information about Vivli, including current Vivli metrics and members, is available at https://vivli.org (accessed February 10, 2020).

[3] At the time of the workshop there were 21 members of Vivli, including industry, academia, nonprofit funders and foundations, and patient/disease advocacy organizations. See https://vivli.org/members/ourmembers (accessed March 2, 2020).

[4] A printable brochure of the 2015 IOM report recommendation for when to share specific types of data is available at http://nationalacademies.org/hmd/~/media/Files/Report%20 Files/2015/SharingData/RAAG_ShareData_Print.pdf (accessed February 10, 2020).

Challenges

Li described some of the challenges for the Vivli data contributors and data users. The anonymization of contributed datasets can be challenging, especially for rare disease datasets. Sharing large datasets, often including tens of thousands of patients, also presents challenges, especially when the data include imaging. In response to a question, Li said that Vivli can offer solutions to researchers facing governance hurdles, such as when researchers want to share, but their institutions are reluctant.

One challenge for data users is the siloing of data sources. Some, but not all, of the data might be submitted to Vivli, with some data remaining elsewhere (e.g., within the institution). Li said this challenge is frustrating for users and limits analysis. Another challenge is the heterogeneity of data formats. Li added that data supply and demand are not balanced, and Vivli is working to increase awareness of this rich data resource and to raise the number of users.

Lessons Learned

Li concluded with three lessons learned from the Vivli experience:

1. **Balancing flexibility and harmonization.** A data-sharing platform, Li noted, must be both *flexible* in meeting the needs of its individual users (e.g., in respecting the data contributor's governance, review process, data types, and tools), and *harmonious* in providing the best user experience (e.g., by developing master DUAs to improve efficiency).
2. **Addressing the complexities of sharing individual participant data.** The technical and governance aspects of data sharing are complicated, Li said. Platforms need to engage stakeholders to effectively address these challenges. She observed that in many cases, potential data contributors are not deciding which platform to use to share but are deciding whether to share or not. The challenge for platforms is to present sharing as the compelling option.
3. **Enabling data sharing.** The role of a nonprofit organization that manages a platform is to enable data sharing by, for example, providing training and resources, lowering cost barriers, and providing digital object identifiers. A nonprofit platform cannot influence or incentivize data sharing. "The broader research ecosystem of funders, academia, and publishers holds the levers to reward investigators for sharing data for the public good," Li said.

THE YODA PROJECT

Joseph Ross, Professor of Medicine and Public Health, Yale School of Medicine

The Yale University Open Data Access (YODA) Project was launched in 2011 with the intent of making research data available to the broader scientific community.[5] In 2014, the YODA Project formed a partnership with Johnson & Johnson to facilitate sharing of clinical trial data for the company's pharmaceutical products (including data from legacy trials), as well as devices and diagnostics, Ross said. Policies and procedures for data access were developed with input from the YODA Project steering committee, stakeholders, and the public.

Ross outlined the guiding principles of the YODA Project:

- Promote the sharing of clinical research data to advance science and improve public health and health care.
- Promote the responsible conduct of research.
- Ensure good stewardship of clinical research data by external investigators.
- Protect the rights of research participants.

The YODA Model

Researchers can search for trials by National Clinical Trial number or can filter the repository entries by criteria such as product or generic name, therapeutic area, condition, or enrollment parameters. Information provided for each trial includes general information about the product and trial and (when available) links to the Clinical Study Report Summary, the ClinicalTrials.gov trial record, the primary citation, study data specifications, and the annotated case report form.

When secondary data users identify a trial of interest, Ross explained, they must apply for access to the data, while listing all investigators and their affiliations and funding and including a narrative summary, a public abstract, and a detailed proposal for the intended research. Ross said that the detailed proposal facilitates accountability and integrity as the broader research community can later compare the submitted request with the subsequent findings or publication. Data requesters must also submit a timeline and a dissemination plan and complete DUA training, Ross added.

[5] Further information about the YODA project, including the data request process and current metrics, can be found at https://yoda.yale.edu (accessed February 10, 2020) and in Ross et al. (2018). The YODA Project is funded by a research grant through Yale from Johnson & Johnson and was formerly funded by Medtronic.

The YODA Project completes the process of reviewing applications for scientific merit within about 2 weeks. Proposals are reviewed to ensure that the scientific purpose of the work is clearly described and that it is possible to conduct the proposed study using the requested data. In addition, the review verifies that "the data requested will be used to generate or materially enhance generalizable scientific and/or medical knowledge to inform science and public health," Ross said. The data generator partner reviews the proposal simultaneously to determine whether they can make the data available. The data generator partner's due diligence includes assessment of the appropriateness of the requested data for the proposed research, and also considers whether patient privacy will be protected and if similar research studies have used the same data being requested.

After the data request is approved and the DUA is signed, the investigators can access the data on a secure platform via a virtual private network, which Ross said protects patient privacy and helps prevent further distribution of the data. He added that DUA negotiations add the most time to the request process, often taking 3 months or more to come to an agreement.

YODA Project Metrics

Since forming its partnership with Johnson & Johnson during the last quarter of 2014, YODA has made data available from 350 trials for request, 75 percent of which have been requested for use, Ross said. About 90 percent of the investigators making data requests are from academia, he said, and requests have come from around the world. The median number of trials requested per data request is three. Of 134 data request applications submitted, 87 percent (117) were approved, 3 percent are under review, and 10 percent have been withdrawn or closed because the data are not in the repository or cannot be made available for use (e.g., unable to adequately deidentify). He added that no request has yet been rejected. About 80 percent of the requests required administrative revisions, and about 30 percent required scientific revision prior to approval. Ross illustrated the status of the data requests over the previous 5 years (see Figure 3-1). He clarified that the studies indicated in orange have not pursued publication, but the results are reported on the YODA Project website. All requests for data are publicly posted on the YODA Project website after the DUA is signed, regardless of status, Ross said. It is not expected that all requests will lead to a publication, he said, but added that 31 manuscripts have been submitted for publication thus far, of which 26 have been published, and there have also been 26 posters and conference presentations. Ross highlighted several of the key publications that used data made available through the YODA

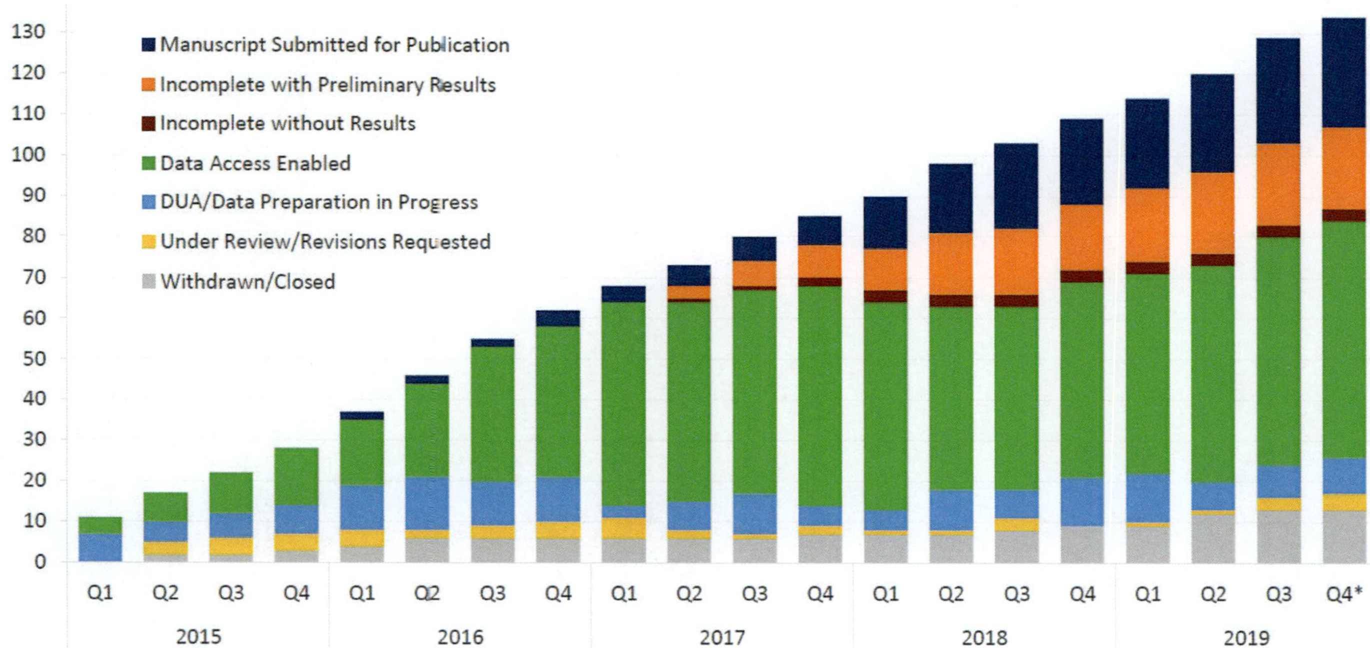

FIGURE 3-1 Status of data requests by quarter (as of November 1, 2019).
NOTE: DUA = data use agreement.
SOURCE: As presented by Joseph Ross, November 18, 2019.

Project (see Corbett et al., 2017; Mbuagbaw et al., 2019). More than half of the data requests indicate that the purpose of the analysis is meta-analysis or to answer a new question. Other responses include clinical prediction, validation, statistical methods, clinical trial methods, pilot research, comparison group, or other. Ross noted that investigators can indicate more than one purpose of the analysis.

Lessons Learned

In conclusion, Ross said that as a result of the YODA Project, "there have now been numerous studies that might not otherwise have been feasible to pursue, some of which have impacted health policy and guidelines." The platform has also enabled researchers to directly collaborate with the original investigators at Johnson & Johnson. Importantly, Ross said, Johnson & Johnson now conducts clinical trials with the intent that the data will be shared (i.e., planning in advance for data sharing).

With regard to concerns about potential unintended consequences, Ross said that "replication studies have supported, not undermined, the original study, there have been no instances of patient privacy breaches, no publications of spurious safety findings that received unwarranted attention or disrupted patient care, and no data have been used for commercial or litigious purposes."

Ross highlighted several areas where attention is needed to better reap the rewards of data sharing. He reiterated the point by Li that there is a need to raise researcher awareness of the available data resources. He also noted that many researchers requesting data do not have expertise in using clinical data. It would be helpful for analyses if older trial data could be made available in a contemporary format and if sponsors adopted uniform data standards for current trials. Ross additionally noted a need to address sustainability and the costs of data sharing.

SOAR

Frank Rockhold, Professor of Biostatistics and Bioinformatics, Duke Clinical Research Institute

The SOAR platform is a collaboration among the DCRI, academia, and industry that is intended to facilitate open and transparent sharing of clinical research data among investigators, data scientists, and statisticians to inform and accelerate science for the benefit of human health.[6]

[6] Further information about the SOAR platform is available at https://dcri.org/our-work/analytics-and-data-science/data-sharing (accessed February 10, 2020).

BOX 3-1
Goals and Principles of Open Science at the Duke University School of Medicine

Advance Science
- Answer new questions
- Combine data to increase its power
- Avoid duplication of effort
- Foster new connections and collaborations

Improve Research Integrity
- Validate original analyses
- Promote transparency and trustworthiness

Principles
- Facilitate appropriate access
- Ensure appropriate governance
- Maintain data utility
- Share results (and data) from secondary analyses
- Acknowledge and provide academic credit for those who share original data

SOURCES: Rockhold presentation, November 18, 2019; adapted from the Duke Roadmap for Open Science, available at https://medschool.duke.edu/about-us/news-and-communications/med-school-blog/introducing-duke-school-medicine-roadmap-open-science (accessed February 10, 2020).

Rockhold explained that one goal of the platform is to facilitate progress on data sharing in the academic world, as much of the clinical trial data sharing thus far has been done by industry. He outlined the Duke University School of Medicine's principles for open science and data sharing (see Box 3-1) and emphasized that there are active discussions regarding the final principles about how to provide proper academic credit to researchers who share original data.

The SOAR Model

Although SOAR also serves as an independent review panel for clinical trial datasets being shared by industry, specifically Bristol-Myers Squibb (BMS), it contains additional components that make it different from other platforms. For example, SOAR shares the DCRI datasets, including the Duke Cardiac Catheterization Research Dataset and the Duke Cardiac Catheterization Educational Dataset. SOAR also functions as a portal to other datasets, including the Aggregate Analysis of ClinicalTrials.gov database,[7] and datasets that are shared by the National Institutes of Health, the American Heart Association, and others. Rockhold referred participants to his poster for full details about the SOAR platform.[8]

Rockhold briefly described the process for requesting access to BMS clinical trial datasets, which is comparable to that of the other platforms and includes IRP administrative review of proposals, internal review by BMS for availability of the data for sharing, and scientific review by content experts from within Duke. Rockhold described the scientific review as interactive, involving two-way communication between the IRP and the researchers to address concerns and resubmit the proposal.[9] He recalled only one proposal that had been rejected by the IRP thus far, and it was rejected because the proposed study had been done and published by another group. One of the primary reasons the IRP requests additional information or revision is a lack of necessary expertise to conduct the proposed study (e.g., informatics, data scientists, statisticians). In most cases, he said, the investigators add the necessary subject matter experts.

Requests for BMS or Duke data are primarily from academia, with only a small number of requests coming from industry, Rockhold said, noting that sources of requests are similar to those experienced by the YODA project discussed by Ross (see above). He added that there are also about 100 pending requests that will be reviewed after the data become available for sharing, as noted above, 2 years from "database lock," a step in clinical research that limits unauthorized modifications to clinical trial data.

Challenges

There seems to be little overlap between those who contribute data and those who seek to access it, Rockhold observed. He reiterated that most of the data sharing is being done by industry while most of the data requesters are from academia, which he noted are two scientific communities that do not necessarily speak the same scientific language. Persistent barriers to data sharing include patient privacy concerns, costs, inoperability/lack of data standards, and data integrity. Rockhold said the challenge is to demonstrate that the benefits of data sharing outweigh the risks (see Figure 3-2).

---

7 A project of the Clinical Trials Transformation Initiative to improve public access to aggregate data in ClinicalTrials.gov. See https://aact.ctti-clinicaltrials.org (accessed March 2, 2020).

8 Available on the workshop webpage, http://nationalacademies.org/hmd/Activities/Research/DrugForum/2019-Nov-18.aspx (accessed February 10, 2020), under the Attachments menu.

9 The review criteria are available at https://dcri.org/our-work/analytics-and-data-science/data-sharing/bms-studies (accessed February 10, 2020).

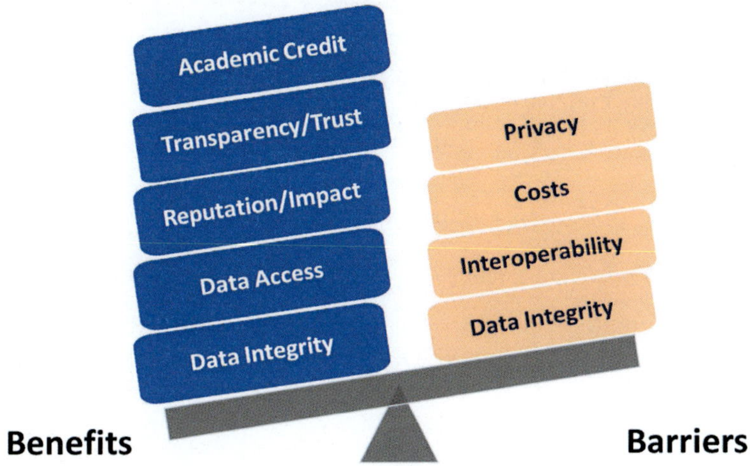

FIGURE 3-2 The desired future state is one in which the benefits of data sharing clearly outweigh the barriers.
SOURCE: As presented by Frank Rockhold, November 18, 2019.

Rockhold suggested that the process of data sharing will become a bit easier when there is greater overlap between the communities (i.e., when more data contributors are also data users and vice versa). With a better understanding of each other's perspective, data generators might collect and steward data in a way that better facilitates sharing, and data users might be able to propose secondary analyses that make the best use of the available data.

CLINICALSTUDYDATAREQUEST.COM

Scott Shaunessy, Co-Founder and Chair, ClinicalStudyDataRequest.com

CSDR was launched in 2013 as a clinical trial data-sharing initiative of GlaxoSmithKline, and then relaunched as a multi-sponsor site in 2014 with the addition of Roche, Novartis, and Boehringer Ingelheim. As one of the first data-sharing platforms, the initial focus of the platform was to protect data from misuse, Shaunessy said. The platform is constantly evolving, he said, and in recent years CSDR has worked with technology partners, including SAS,[10] to provide analytics tools and to make

[10] SAS develops advanced technology and analytics solutions. See https://www.sas.com/en_us/home.html (accessed March 2, 2020).

the platform experience more "researcher centric." Shaunessy focused his panel remarks on challenges and solutions as he said CSDR essentially works the same way as the other three platforms presented (see above), and the metrics for CSDR were already discussed by Kochhar (see Chapter 2).[11]

Challenges and Solutions

Establishing a Truly Independent IRP

An early challenge, Shaunessy said, was that the IRP was not seen as truly independent because CSDR and the sponsor companies selected the IRP. To remedy this, Wellcome Trust was approached in 2015 about serving as the secretariat for the IRP (as discussed by Kochhar in Chapter 2). The IRP is now a rotating group of five members, with additional therapeutic area experts engaged by Wellcome Trust as needed.

Transparency and Metrics

Another challenge is ensuring transparency, and Shaunessy said that CSDR began to publish metrics on the website as soon as possible after launch and updates the numbers quarterly. He referred participants to his poster and the CSDR website for more information.[12]

Speed to Research

Shaunessy reiterated that a current focus is on making the platform more useful for researchers, and one element of doing so is reducing the time from request to data access. A range of factors can cause delays, but he said that "the single biggest obstacle has been the data-sharing agreement." CSDR worked with all member companies to develop a single data sharing agreement that he said is favorable to the researchers' institutions. However, he said that institutions still seek to negotiate aspects of the agreement. In an ongoing effort to increase transparency, Shaunessy noted that one of the metrics now being posted on the website is the "cycle time" from initial proposal to start of research.

[11] Further information about the CSDR platform is available at https://www.clinicalstudydatarequest.com (accessed February 10, 2020).

[12] The poster is available on the workshop webpage, http://nationalacademies.org/hmd/Activities/Research/DrugForum/2019-Nov-18.aspx (accessed February 10, 2020), under the Attachments menu.

Sharing Data Between Other Multi-Sponsor and Single-Sponsor Platforms

Another challenge for researchers is attempting to conduct a study across multiple clinical trials and across multiple companies when the data are housed in different data-sharing platforms, company systems, and/or academic institutions. In many cases, researchers must resort to making multiple separate data requests and then conducting parallel research projects, which they must then interpret and attempt to combine the results.

The next step for data sharing is for platforms and clinical trial sponsors to work together to identify solutions that allow secondary analyses to combine data across platforms. "The result will be better research, better outcomes, and the advancement of human health," Shaunessy concluded.

Another challenge raised by Colin Baigent, deputy director of the Clinical Trial Service and Epidemiological Studies Units at Oxford University, is that data-sharing platforms, in their current form, do not readily enable sophisticated statistical meta-analysis, which requires holding a local copy of the data from multiple trials and sponsors. Therefore, his approach has been to try to obtain data directly from the originator (i.e., keep a local copy of the data with which to work). Shaunessy agreed and said the mindset about directly sharing data is shifting, and he said he was aware of one CSDR member company that is planning to directly share data.

4

Striking a Balance Between Benefit/Value and Risk/Cost

Highlights of Key Points Made by Individual Speakers

- Data sharing can uncover issues (e.g., error, fraud), enable alternative analysis approaches, lead to new insights, generate additional publications, and facilitate new collaborations. (DeMets)
- Phase 3 clinical trials generally collect much more data than are ever used, which creates challenges for documentation and storage. Despite the volume of data, trial documentation often lacks key details needed for successful reproduction of the analyses. (DeMets)
- Clinical investigators tend to collect as much information as possible because they do not want to reach the end of the study and find that an important data element was not collected. (Drazen)
- The new generation of medical practitioners has expertise in data science and can readily use shared clinical trial data to help identify novel findings. Historically, trialists have collaborated primarily with other clinical groups but are now being engaged by data scientists who are interested in conducting independent analyses. (Drazen)
- There is limited information about the attitudes of the general public toward the privacy of health information, but the first users of those data should be the individuals themselves. (Peel)

The third panel to consider the current landscape for clinical trial data sharing and reuse provided stakeholder perspectives on balancing the value and benefits of sharing data with the risks and costs. Or, as expressed by speakers throughout the workshop, "is the juice worth the squeeze?" David DeMets, professor emeritus in the Department of Biostatistics and Biomedical Informatics at the University of Wisconsin, described four case examples of the value that can be derived from data sharing. Jeffrey M. Drazen, *New England Journal of Medicine* group editor, discussed the Systolic Blood Pressure Intervention Trial (SPRINT) Data Analysis Challenge as an example of how clinical trial data can be used to identify new findings of medical importance. Deborah Peel, founder and president of Patient Privacy Rights, discussed public attitudes toward health data privacy. The panel discussion was moderated by Bernard Lo.

DATA ANALYST PERSPECTIVE

David DeMets, Professor Emeritus,
Department of Biostatistics and Biomedical Informatics,
University of Wisconsin

DeMets shared four case examples of the value that can be derived from secondary analysis of shared data, three of which demonstrate how data sharing can uncover issues and provide lessons (e.g., elucidate the impact of methodology on interpretation, identify errors or fraud), and a fourth that led to new insights and additional publications and collaborations.

Data Sharing Can Uncover Issues

Anturane Reinfarction Trial

The Anturane Reinfarction Trial was a randomized controlled trial comparing Anturane (sulfinpyrazone) to placebo for preventing mortality in patients who had experienced myocardial infarction. At the request of the U.S. Food and Drug Administration, DeMets conducted an independent secondary analysis of the trial data, which revealed that not all mortality events had been reported in a 1980 publication on sudden death events during the trial (ART Research Group, 1980; Temple and Pledger, 1980). Participants had been removed from the analysis because it was determined that they were not eligible per the preestablished trial entry criteria (i.e., they should not have been enrolled in the trial). Analyzing the full dataset, including the excluded patients, DeMets found additional mortality events. Taking these additional events into account did not change the overall trends observed with the treatment, DeMets said, but did eliminate the statistical significance. He suggested that this trial "contributed to the concept of intention to treat (ITT) as the primary analysis method." (In an ITT analysis, all participants who are randomized into the trial are included in the analysis of the group into which they were randomized.) This example of a secondary analysis of the data demonstrates how the methods of analysis matter in interpretation.

APPROVe Trial

The Adenomatous Polyp Prevention on Vioxx (APPROVe) Trial was a randomized controlled trial of Vioxx (rofecoxib) versus placebo for the prevention of colon cancer.[1] An analysis published in 2005 suggested that Vioxx was associated with increased cardiovascular events, and the trial was terminated early (Bresalier et al., 2005). Per the protocol, participants were followed for 14 days after discontinuation of therapy. After the trial was terminated, DeMets and colleagues conducted a follow-up analysis of cardiovascular outcomes in patients for an additional year after termination of treatment and found that participants had an increased rate of select cardiovascular events (Baron et al., 2008). This secondary analysis allows the impact of informative censoring[2] to be shown. In other words, "off drug does not mean off study," DeMets said.

Genomic Predictors of Cancer: The Duke Translational Omics Case

In the third example described by DeMets, secondary analysis of shared data uncovered fraud and led to the retraction of publications. Duke University researchers Anil Potti and Joseph Nevins published several high-profile papers describing genomic predictors of cancer risk and therapeutic response, and these genomic predictors were subsequently used in Duke clinical trials. However, statisticians at MD Anderson were unable to reproduce the Duke researchers' results. Further analysis of data shared by Duke revealed numerous concerns with both the data and the analysis (Baggerly and Coombes, 2009). Ultimately, DeMets said, the work by Potti and Nevins was shown to be fraudulent, and many of the papers were withdrawn. He referred participants to

[1] See https://clinicaltrials.gov/ct2/show/NCT00282386 (accessed March 2, 2020).

[2] Censored data are data that are outside of an established boundary or threshold and are therefore not fully elucidated (in this case, the censored data are the cardiovascular events that occurred beyond the 14-day follow-up period). Informative censoring is when clinical trial participants are lost to follow-up because of study-related reasons (in this case, the lack of data collection beyond 14 days after discontinuation of treatment is a result of the predefined study protocol).

the 2012 Institute of Medicine (IOM) consensus study report *Evolution of Translational Omics: Lessons Learned and the Path Forward* for more detailed information about the case (IOM, 2012b).

Data Sharing Can Lead to Additional Publications and Collaborations

The COMPANION Trial

The Comparison of Medical Therapy, Pacing, and Defibrillation in Heart Failure (COMPANION) Trial was a randomized controlled clinical trial of a pacemaker, with or without defibrillator, versus optimal pharmacologic treatment in patients with heart failure.[3] The study found that a pacemaker, alone and with a defibrillator, provided significant survival benefit over medical therapy (Bristow et al., 2004).

DeMets, the lead statistician for the study, had the opportunity to revisit the data a decade after the primary and secondary papers were published and develop additional manuscripts for publication. DeMets set out to reproduce the original 2004 study prior to conducting additional analyses and faced several barriers. Finding the data from a decade ago was difficult (data are often migrated to a different system), and the dataset he first retrieved and used was not the final file that had been used for the published paper. When the correct documentation was ultimately retrieved, it lacked key details needed to reproduce the study, and the software used a decade prior had changed, he said. After finally reproducing the original paper, DeMets was able to publish several additional analyses and said that several more are in progress.

DeMets and Lo have previously published on the need to promote collaboration between the original clinical investigators and the researchers conducting secondary analyses (Lo and DeMets, 2016), and DeMets said he engaged members of the COMPANION Trial steering committee. He observed that being offered co-authorship seemed to help reduce their resistance to data sharing and secondary analysis. DeMets also engaged new cardiovascular investigators (i.e., medical fellows, younger faculty). Together, this approach allowed the authors to gain new insights into the use of pacemakers and defibrillators in heart failure patients, he said.

Reflections on the Benefits and Costs of Data Sharing

Speaking from his perspective as a data analyst, DeMets reflected on the potential benefits and costs associated with data sharing. Archiving a complete clinical trial data file in a form and level of detail sufficient for

[3] See https://clinicaltrials.gov/ct2/show/NCT00180258 (accessed March 2, 2020).

future use requires significant effort and cost. Despite one's best efforts and intentions, it is likely that details needed to reproduce the findings are not documented sufficiently, he said. Secondary analyses can catch errors and fraud which, although infrequent, are important. Secondary analyses also allow for the investigation of alternative analysis approaches. Importantly, "data sharing can produce further research and maximize the benefit of the trial," DeMets said. In closing, he said, "Phase 3 randomized controlled trials collect more data than are ever typically used," which creates challenges for documentation and storage. He advocated for designing simpler trials that minimize the amount of data that are documented and stored and suggested concentrating data-sharing resources on pivotal Phase 3 clinical trials over earlier phase studies.

PUBLISHER PERSPECTIVE

Jeffrey M. Drazen, New England Journal of Medicine *Group Editor*

Drazen discussed some of the concerns about data sharing and secondary analysis raised by three key stakeholder groups: clinical trialists, participants, and data scientists; he further presented the SPRINT Data Analysis Challenge as an example of how clinical trial data can be used to identify new findings of medical importance. He also took the opportunity to respond to the comment by DeMets (see above) about the vast amount of data collected in Phase 3 clinical trials. Drazen said that investigators tend to collect as much information as possible because they fear reaching the end of the study and realizing an important data element was not collected.

Stakeholder Concerns

Clinical Trialists

Historically, clinical trialists have essentially owned their trial data by default and have collaborated almost exclusively with other clinical groups studying the same disease area, Drazen said. Around the mid-2000s, the emergence of data science and the ability to store large volumes of data led to data scientists requesting access to clinical trial data to conduct independent analyses. Sophisticated statistical packages are now available, and early-career scientists are adept at writing code for data analysis.

Drazen explained that clinical trialists are invested in formulating a sound clinical question, collecting data, analyzing the data according to a preestablished statistical analysis plan, and drawing a conclusion to answer the clinical question. In general, any deviation from the established clinical protocol is avoided, as it can introduce bias. "When you hunt for signals, you find them," Drazen said, and when health and lives are at stake, it is essential to be sure that the signals identified, whether positive or negative, are real. Therefore, clinical trialists are concerned about drawing clinically directive conclusions from post hoc analyses. Post hoc analyses are instead used for informing the design of the next clinical trial. Drazen noted that there are many examples where a strong signal that was apparent in the dataset was not borne out in a subsequent clinical trial. Another concern is that conducting a trial takes a lot of time and effort, and trialists want to reap the academic reward for their work, one form of which is publications in journals.

Participants

A primary concern for trial participants is privacy. As discussed by Moses Taylor, Jr. (see Chapter 2), patients want their data to be widely but responsibly used, Drazen said. The data users, he said, need to define how the data will be used and to ensure responsible use. A question for consideration is who should be allowed to use the data? For example, Drazen said, if participants could potentially be identified from the data, should the study be subject to institutional review board review to ensure that data are not misused?

Data Scientists

Data scientists believe transparency and data sharing can promote public confidence in clinical research, Drazen said (e.g., through the reproduction or replication of studies). When data are not made public, there can be mistrust of the research and study outcomes. Importantly, secondary analysis of shared data by data scientists can reveal new information and ideas that can advance human health, he said.

SPRINT Data Analysis Challenge

Drazen elaborated on SPRINT, introduced by Taylor (see Chapter 2). Planning for SPRINT began in 2009 with the trial anticipated to run until 2017. The study compared more intensive blood pressure control (lowering to at or below 120 mm Hg) to standard blood pressure control (lowering to at or below 140 mm Hg) in nearly 10,000 patients age 50 years or older with increased cardiovascular risk and systolic blood pressure between 130 and 180 mm Hg.

In 2015, SPRINT was stopped early when the Data and Safety Monitoring Board (DSMB) observed the significant positive outcomes associated with intensive intervention (SPRINT Research Group, 2015). Drazen relayed that the case rate of high blood pressure complications (e.g., heart attack, stroke) was significantly lower in the intensive treatment group versus the standard treatment group (16 cases per 1,000 versus 21 cases per 1,000, respectively).

Following the announcement by the National Institutes of Health (NIH) that SPRINT was being stopped early due to the important positive findings, Harlan Krumholz and Eric Topol opined in *The New York Times* that the data should be made public immediately, which was prior to the peer-reviewed publication of the final results.[4] Drazen said that, in his opinion, the clinical investigators know the data best and deserve the opportunity to analyze it, and report on it on behalf of the study participants who have put themselves at risk for the study, before making the dataset public. He noted that the study results were published just 2 months later.

The dataset underlying the findings presented in the 2015 SPRINT publication was released 1 year later. To explore how clinical trial data can be used to identify new findings of medical importance, the *New England Journal of Medicine* sponsored the SPRINT Data Analysis Challenge.[5] Of 279 requests for access to the data that were received from around the world, 218 advanced to a qualifying round designed to demonstrate that the requester had the necessary statistical skillset to use the data. Two hundred research groups advanced to the challenge round, and 143 entered the final round. Drazen reported that, among the three finalists, one group of mid-career researchers said they spent several weeks deriving their response to the challenge round (and required a hint from the Challenge), while a group of second-year medical students said they obtained the correct answer in about 20 minutes. The difference, Drazen observed, was that the younger-generation researchers had developed the skills to code their own statistical analysis packages as needed. The new generation entering medicine has expertise in data science, he said, and can use shared clinical trial data to identify novel findings. Drazen also noted that after the dataset was made public, errors were found by others; although none impacted the outcome, they were corrected. He concluded that there are many positive aspects of having many different people analyze clinical trial data, but there are also challenges, such as the cost and effort to facilitate sharing. To encourage both data sharing and secondary analysis, it is important to demonstrate the value that can be obtained, and examples are needed of how secondary analysis has led to behavioral change that impacted health as confirmed by another clinical trial.

---

[4] See https://www.nytimes.com/2015/09/18/opinion/dont-delay-news-of-medical-breakthroughs.html (accessed February 10, 2020).

[5] See https://challenge.nejm.org/pages/home (accessed February 10, 2020).

PATIENT PERSPECTIVE

Deborah Peel, Founder and President, Patient Privacy Rights

Peel, a practicing physician and Freudian psychoanalyst, spoke from her perspective as a patient privacy rights advocate. She discussed public attitudes toward the privacy of health information in general (i.e., not specific to clinical trials). She emphasized that there is a universal human right to privacy.[6] In Europe, she said, "privacy means the right to self-determination, autonomy, respect, and control over personal information." She noted that there is not an established definition of this privacy in the United States. Furthermore, she referred participants to a section of the 2002 Amended Health Insurance Portability and Accountability Act Privacy Rule that she said actually strips individuals of their right to control their own health data (67 *Federal Register* 53,183). Specifically, Peel said that "covered entities can use and disclose information for treatment, payment, and health care operations." She expressed concern that most uses could be deemed to fall into those categories, and that health data are being treated as a "corporate asset." She also pointed out that the flow of personal data—or where and with whom the data are shared—is not mapped, making the environment difficult to understand.

Peel mentioned two current examples of sharing of real-world health data. Project Nightingale by Google is collecting patient health data through an agreement with a large health system and without the knowledge of patients or providers.[7] Apple is now involved in medical research by, for example, enabling clinical research recruiting through a phone app and using new technologies, such as the Apple Watch that can collect health data, to conduct research in new ways.

Patient Attitudes About Privacy

The research on the public's attitudes about privacy and the use of their health data is very limited, Peel said. Although there have been surveys of clinical trial participants (e.g., Mello et al., 2018), there are few, if any, published surveys of the general public. She mentioned one survey done in 2007 by Alan Westin at the request of an IOM consensus

[6] This is mentioned in Article 12 of the Universal Declaration of Human Rights. See https://www.un.org/en/universal-declaration-human-rights (accessed March 2, 2020).

[7] Peel listed several recent news articles as background on Project Nightingale, including https://www.wsj.com/articles/google-s-secret-project-nightingale-gathers-personal-health-data-on-millions-of-americans-11573496790 (accessed February 10, 2020), and on the Apple initiative, https://www.nytimes.com/2019/11/14/technology/apple-harvard-health-studies.html (accessed February 10, 2020).

study committee to inform their work. Peel highlighted Westin's finding that "only 1 percent of the public would ever agree to unfettered access to their records without consent." In a 2016 survey of U.S. consumer attitudes toward health information technology, 89 percent of respondents said they withheld health information from their health care providers.[8] There is public distrust in the system, which impacts the quality of data in the health system, which can impact health outcomes, she continued.

Peel noted that there is some movement toward ensuring that the public's health data remain private. As mentioned, the Apple initiative is enabling researchers to reach out to members of the public who are interested in participating in research. Apple has assured Apple Watch users that their health data will never be shared by Apple or its partners without their consent. Peel suggested the need for something similar to a "nutrition label" for smartphone and device apps that would provide users with information on the level of privacy protection afforded them.[9] Smartphones and wearables can now collect large volumes of data about an individual's health as well as many other relevant parameters, and Peel said the first users of those data should be the individuals themselves. She referred participants to the work of Alex "Sandy" Pentland of the Massachusetts Institute of Technology and his "New Deal on Data" for further discussion of an individual's ownership of their own data and control of the data flow.[10]

DISCUSSION

Metrics of Value

Colin Baigent asked about the metrics available to determine whether the value created by the sharing of clinical trial data is worth the costs. Quantitative metrics of the impacts and outputs of data sharing are needed to make the business case for the allocation of resources to support sharing. He said he had searched and found that the publications arising directly from work done by the three SPRINT Data Analysis Challenge winners had been cited only 14 times, which he said did not seem to demonstrate sufficient value for the effort.[11]

---

[8] Peel referred participants to https://blackbookmarketresearch.newswire.com/news/healthcares-digital-divide-widens-black-book-consumer-survey-18432252 (accessed February 10, 2020).

[9] Further information about the proposed label is available at https://papers.ssrn.com/sol3/papers.cfm?abstract_id=3439701 (accessed February 10, 2020).

[10] See https://hd.media.mit.edu/wef_globalit.pdf (accessed February 10, 2020).

[11] See https://www.nature.com/articles/s41746-019-0156-3 (accessed March 31, 2020); https://www.ncbi.nlm.nih.gov/pubmed/31067189 (accessed March 31, 2020); and https://journals.plos.org/plosmedicine/article?id=10.1371/journal.pmed.1002410 (accessed March 31, 2020).

Drazen recalled that, in the mid-1990s, NIH and Wellcome Trust required their grantees involved in the Human Genome Project to deposit DNA sequence data in a public database. He noted that opinion in the genetics community was divided, with some supporting the sharing of sequences to advance the field and others opposing the requirement to give away the results of their hard work. Today, he continued, it is standard practice to deposit sequences into the National Center for Biotechnology Information database of Genotypes and Phenotypes (dbGaP)[12] and other databases. Researchers worldwide can access the shared sequence data to inform the development of experimental questions and study design.

With this in mind, Drazen suggested that the number of peer-reviewed publications associated with shared clinical trial data might not be the ideal metric of the value of clinical trial data sharing. Like sequence data, clinical trial data might be accessed to inform study design or help conceptualize questions, which he said could reduce the need for putting patients at risk for exploratory studies. Baigent agreed that citation metrics are not the only option. Both agreed that the challenge is how to measure uses of shared data that do not directly result in a publication. Lo added that there might be other unpublished uses of trial data and emphasized the importance of data-sharing platforms asking users who accesses the data, what they are using it for, and whether the data were helpful for their task.

Matthew Sydes, professor of clinical trials and methodology at the University College London, observed that SPRINT was a large trial of 10,000 participants, resulting in a vast amount of data. He asked whether there is a minimum enrollment size at which trials have more utility for data sharing and for analysis challenges such as that done with the SPRINT data. DeMets agreed that, in general, it is most efficient to target resources and efforts toward shared data from well-powered studies. Drazen cautioned against defining which trials are important to share based on enrollment size. A large trial can have no relevant findings or impact, and a small trial can change clinical practice. It is not possible to know until the end. Data from trials that could potentially change clinical thinking should be shared, Drazen noted.

Combining Data Across Trials and Platforms

Alex Sherman highlighted the importance of being able to merge and harmonize data from multiple clinical trials.[13] He mentioned two such

[12] For information on dbGaP, see https://www.ncbi.nlm.nih.gov/gap (accessed March 2, 2020).

[13] Also discussed by Shaunessy in Chapter 3.

existing models of data sharing. The Critical Path Institute, for example, has been facilitating data sharing for more than a decade, merging data from multiple clinical trials in a disease area or across multiple diseases.[14] There is also the amyotrophic lateral sclerosis (ALS or Lou Gehrig's disease) dataset that merges harmonized data from 23 ALS clinical trials. He said that 1,500 researchers from 64 countries have used the data, leading to multiple publications. He also mentioned an ALS crowdsourcing challenge in which 1,100 researchers participated. Lo suggested that perhaps the time has come for platforms that facilitate sharing of single studies to combine their resources and enable researchers to combine data and conduct analyses across platforms.

Informed Consent for Data Sharing

Sherman noted the need for standardized data-sharing practices and standardized legal documents. He said the informed consent form for all clinical trials his institution conducts includes participant consent that their data will be used for any medical research purpose. Peel raised concern that a choice between not sharing one's data or giving blanket consent to share one's data "forever in the future without asking the person again" is not a meaningful choice and contributes to patient distrust in the health system. Taylor said that, as a trial participant, "as long as I am aware that the data are going to be shared responsibly and I agree to be in the trial, I have given up the right to control those data. I am doing it voluntarily because I can see the benefit of giving up that right for my future health." He said he understood that other trial participants might not want to sign away their privacy rights for the future, but he said people can also choose not to participate in the trial.

Sherman observed that participant willingness to share can be dependent on the disease, and that those with rare diseases are often very willing to share their data to facilitate medical advances. Drazen agreed that patients with rare or life-threatening conditions are often willing to take on greater risk for incremental progress. However, he suggested that people might not be willing to put their privacy at risk for a more common and relatively mild condition (e.g., hypertension). Sherman noted that there is greater risk of deidentification of data in trials for rare conditions, especially if the participants have been enrolled in multiple trials.

DeMets supported participants' rights but added his concern that secondary analyses can be subject to bias depending on which partici-

[14] See https://c-path.org (accessed February 10, 2020).

pants consent or decline to share their data. The primary publication would include the full trial population. However, downstream analyses are impacted by if—and the extent to which—participants have consented to sharing of their data.

5

Data Interoperability and Platform Usability

Highlights of Key Points Made by Individual Speakers

- Data interoperability and platform usability are hampered by insufficient data standardization and collection, and lack of external validity of trial samples. (Hawk)
- Data sharing prior to trial completion and pooling of data across studies can amplify potential safety signals. (Hawk)
- Challenges that researchers face when attempting individual participant data (IPD) meta-analysis include lack of IPD availability, cross-platform incompatibility, and timeframe and practicality issues. (Tianjing Li)
- There is a need for a "single, searchable database that catalogs all IPD available across different platforms," and a mechanism to allow data merging across platforms. (Tianjing Li)
- Platforms generally rely on data providers for data quality assurance, and providers depend on platforms to control data access; there are challenges to be addressed on both sides. (Louv)
- Even within a platform there can be interoperability challenges across the datasets for a given study. Imaging and genomic datasets, for example, are often collected by specialty laboratories that have different data structures, data stewards, and data deidentification schemes than those for other clinical data (e.g., outcomes). (Louv)

The next workshop panel considered the key challenges of data interoperability and platform usability in the context of three case examples. Ernest Hawk, vice president and head of the Division of Cancer Prevention and Population Sciences at MD Anderson, discussed issues of data interoperability and platform usability in the context of cancer prevention trials. Tianjing Li, associate professor at the University of Colorado Denver, described an example of an unsuccessful attempt to conduct an individual patient data network meta-analysis (IPD-NMA). Bill Louv, president of Project Data Sphere, discussed Project Data Sphere as an example of an open-access, data-sharing model and described some of the challenges faced. The session was moderated by Timothy Coetzee, chief advocacy, services, and research officer at the National Multiple Sclerosis Society, and Dina Paltoo, assistant director of Policy Development at the National Library of Medicine at the National Institutes of Health.

WORKING WITH POPULATION DATA

Ernest Hawk, Vice President and Head,
Division of Cancer Prevention and Population Sciences, MD Anderson

Hawk discussed issues of data interoperability and platform usability in the context of cancer prevention trials. He shared three case examples illustrating (1) the value of collecting "the right data" in a standardized form that enables both primary and secondary analyses, (2) the importance of external validity of the trial sample, and (3) the significance of governance and data sharing prior to trial conclusion to enable safety assessment.

Data Standardization and Collection

Data standardization and collection in cancer prevention trials are often insufficient, Hawk said. Standardized questionnaires are not used for data collection, and there is no systematic collection of data on either exposure across the life span or concomitant medication use. Data on concomitant medications are valuable, he explained, because there is a lack of directed investment in drug development for cancer prevention, and insights about preventive medications have been largely serendipitous. Behavioral data are often not collected, and there is also the challenge of incorporating data from mHealth (mobile phone apps and wearables) observations.

Hawk discussed tobacco use as a case example. For more than 50 years, tobacco use has been associated with a range of adverse health consequences, including cancer and cancer-related outcomes. In addition, he said, tobacco use reduces cancer treatment efficacy, and tobacco users experience more significant adverse effects of treatments (e.g., second primary tumors, treatment-related toxicities and morbidities) than former tobacco users or those who never used tobacco. Despite the known negative consequences of tobacco use on cancer outcomes, information about tobacco use has not been systematically collected from participants during oncology clinical trials (Gritz et al., 2005).

A study published in 2012 found that about one-third of trials in the National Cancer Institute's (NCI's) Clinical Trials Cooperative Group Program[1] had assessed tobacco use upon enrollment of participants, less than 5 percent assessed tobacco use during the course of the trial, and none of the trials asked if tobacco users were interested in quitting, Hawk reported. Less than 3 percent of the trials assessed secondhand smoke at enrollment. Any tobacco use data that were collected, he said, were not captured in a standardized form (Peters et al., 2012).

To help address these issues, a task force convened by NCI and the American Association for Cancer Research developed the Cancer Patient Tobacco Use Questionnaire (Land et al., 2016). Hawk said this standardized questionnaire has four core questions to collect a minimal set of data as well as an extended survey, and allows for harmonization of data across studies.

External Validity of Trial Samples

External validity is the extent to which the trial population represents the broader population the trial intends to serve. Hawk pointed out that the underrepresentation of women and minorities in cancer clinical trials persists, despite years of efforts intended to address this issue. Trials also lack diversity in other characteristics that impact cancer outcomes, including genetics and socioeconomic and demographic factors.

Hawk elaborated on recruitment of minority populations to clinical trials, showing recent data on cancer prevalence and cancer trial participation in the United States relative to 2018 U.S. Census data. As shown in Figure 5-1, there is a lack of minority representation in cancer trials. He highlighted several of the barriers to recruitment of underrepresented and minority populations, including lack of awareness of or access to trials, less trust in the health care system, language barriers, and importantly, socioeconomic factors, including lack of insurance coverage (Duma et al., 2018). Great time, effort, and expense go into conducting clinical trials that often do not represent uninsured and under-insured populations in whom cancer diagnoses and poor outcomes are concentrated, Hawk said.

[1] The NCI Clinical Trials Cooperative Group Program is now known as the NCI National Clinical Trials Network. See https://www.cancer.gov/research/areas/clinical-trials/nctn#groups (accessed March 2, 2020).

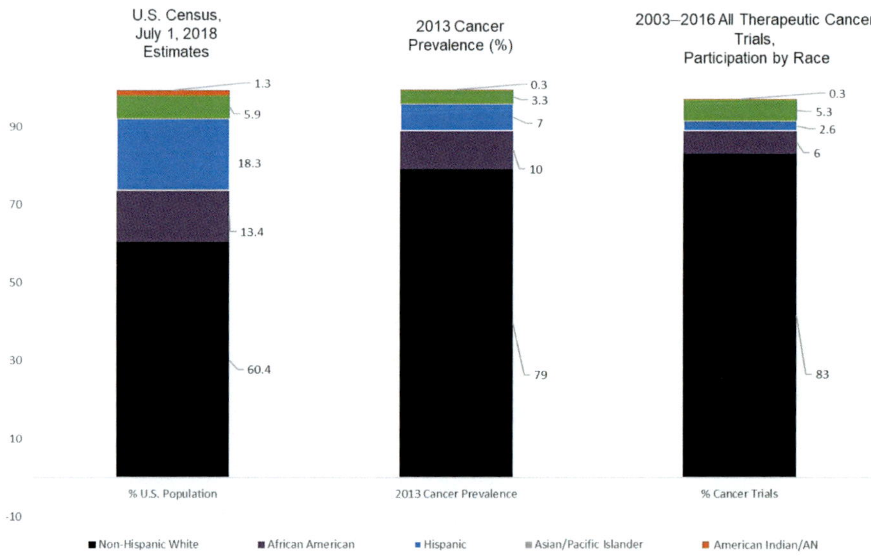

FIGURE 5-1 Minority recruitment to clinical trials.
NOTE: AN = Alaska Native.
SOURCES: As presented by Ernest Hawk, November 18, 2019; based on 2018 U.S. Census data and Duma et al., 2018.

To try to improve minority representation in cancer clinical trials, Regnante and colleagues (2019) looked to U.S. cancer centers of excellence to identify practices that facilitate recruitment and enrollment of racial and ethnic minorities. Examples of strategies identified, Hawk said, included an organizational commitment to diversity, an institutional presence in the community that fosters trust (e.g., community advisory boards, sharing research findings with the community), provider recommendation to a trial, and availability of culturally appropriate materials.

Governance and Data Sharing

Hawk's final example demonstrated the importance of data sharing prior to trial completion to amplify potential safety signals. He described the Adenoma Prevention with Celecoxib (APC) trial of the selective COX-2 inhibitor, celecoxib, for the prevention of colorectal adenomas (Solomon et al., 2005).[2] Although the trial demonstrated efficacy of the intervention, the

[2] See https://clinicaltrials.gov/ct2/show/NCT00005094 (accessed March 2, 2020).

trial was stopped early due to concerns over the potential cardiovascular toxicity of the treatment, Hawk said. To better assess the cardiovascular risk, data were pooled across the APC trial and five other publicly funded, ongoing trials testing celecoxib for different therapeutic or preventive indications (Solomon et al., 2008). Individually, each trial had too few adverse events to assess the cardiovascular risk associated with celecoxib. However, when data were combined, the number of adverse events from the six trials allowed for the elucidation of the dose-related cardiovascular safety concern. Nevertheless, Hawk noted that different baseline data collected in each trial presented a challenge for the analysis.

CHALLENGES FOR META-ANALYSIS

Tianjing Li, Associate Professor, University of Colorado Denver

Li shared a case example of a failed attempt to conduct an individual participant data network meta-analysis. The uniqueness of this approach, she explained, is that the data for the meta-analysis were obtained from data-sharing platforms. As background, she said that greater than 95 percent of published meta-analyses are based on aggregate data, not IPD. Researchers who have done IPD meta-analyses have generally obtained data directly from the trial investigators.

This project was part of the doctoral thesis of Lin Wang, a Ph.D. candidate at Johns Hopkins University, where Li is an adjunct associate professor. Li explained that the student proposed to conduct a systematic review and IPD-NMA on competing treatments for advanced prostate cancer, and to explore whether treatment effect differs by patient characteristics for two tumor types. Wang identified relevant clinical trials that claimed to share IPD on four data-sharing platforms: Vivli, the Yale University Open Data Access (YODA) Project, ClinicalStudyDataRequest.com, and Project Data Sphere.[3] Li said the project faced three key challenges, including IPD availability, cross-platform compatibility, and timeframe and practicality.

Challenges

Lack of IPD Availability

Li explained that, in reviewing the eligible trials for the two tumor types of interest, the student found that IPD were available for only two

[3] For information on Project Data Sphere, see https://projectdatasphere.org/projectdatasphere/html/home (accessed March 2, 2020).

of the six trials for one tumor type, and for one of the seven trials for the other tumor type. According to Li, the trial sponsors gave the student the following reasons for the inability to share IPD:

- The trial was still ongoing or recently had been completed (within 18 or 24 months).
- Regulatory review and approval in the United States and/or European Union were still pending for the product or indication studied.
- "The trial sponsor is not a data contributor, or is a data contributor but the trial of interest is not yet listed, or declined the request because of similar research questions."

The student found that it was relatively easy to find the trial registration numbers, search the data-sharing platforms, identify which trials would share IPD, and submit her data request applications. After that point, however, the process was "out of her control," Li relayed. Although she sent each platform a similar proposal, her experience varied (e.g., some granted permission based on the application as submitted while others required multiple iterations providing additional detail about the research plan).

Cross-Platform Incompatibility

Li said the student also experienced challenges conducting her meta-analysis with IPD obtained from different platforms because of the following:

- Most of the available IPD are not in a downloadable format.
- The data cannot be merged across platforms (cross-platform transmission is prohibited).
- Quality of IPD is inconsistent, metadata are incomplete, and there is a lack of standardization.
- Data of interest might not be in the database.

Timeframe and Practicality

Another challenge the student faced, Li said, was the lag time from the request for IPD to approval by the platform, which ranged from 1 to 8 months. Li pointed out that, after approval, it can take significant time to prepare the dataset for analysis. "Navigating through the different data-sharing models, multiple user accounts, access policies, and procedures … can be challenging for a student or even for a researcher," Li said.

Approaches to Facilitate IPD Meta-Analysis

Li offered her perspective on what is needed to enable meta-analysts to more readily curate data from data-sharing platforms for systematic review. More IPD should be made available on data-sharing platforms, she said. There is also a need for a "single, searchable database that catalogs all IPD available across different platforms," and Li offered the World Health Organization (WHO) International Clinical Trials Registry Platform (ICTRP) as a model.[4] Data-sharing platforms need to have simplified, harmonized, and tiered data request procedures, and she suggested that the institutional review board approval process offers one example of such procedures. A mechanism to allow data merging across different data-sharing platforms is also needed, she said. Data analysts seeking to conduct an IPD meta-analysis "need proper funding, resources, and skills," she continued. In the interim, Li concluded, analysts will need to "consider meta-analysis with both IPD data and aggregate data."

PLATFORM PERSPECTIVE

Bill Louv, President, Project Data Sphere

Louv discussed the unique aspects of the Project Data Sphere open-access, data-sharing platform and described some of the challenges faced.

The Project Data Sphere Model

Project Data Sphere, launched in 2014, is an open-access "digital library-laboratory" created to "broadly share, integrate, and analyze cancer clinical trial data," Louv said. Submission of a research protocol is not required, and access to the full database is provided in about 48–72 hours. Users have free access to SAS analytics software, although Louv noted that most investigators choose to download data and use their own analytical tools. Louv echoed Li's comments and said that "downloading is the only pragmatic way to do meta-analysis across platforms." Thus far, more than 2,500 investigators have collectively made nearly 20,000 data downloads.

The database houses more than 150 datasets from industry and NCI Phase 2 and Phase 3 clinical trials, which include data from more than 125,000 patients. Louv added that about 40 percent of the data are from the experimental arm of the trials and 60 percent are from the comparator arm.

[4] ICTRP is a searchable database of national and regional clinical trial registries. See https://www.who.int/ictrp/search/en (accessed February 10, 2020).

One aspect that sets Project Data Sphere apart is the open-access, data-sharing model (Bertagnolli et al., 2017). Louv observed that YODA and Project Data Sphere are very different models of data sharing, but they have resulted in a similar number of publications, and importantly, there is no evidence of misuse of data or spurious observations made from the data shared on either platform.

Another unique element of Project Data Sphere is its funded research programs (see Figure 5-2). One example, Louv said, uses IPD from comparator arms of small cell lung cancer randomized controlled trials to develop an external control arm. Another program is focused on training machine-learning algorithms to augment radiologist interpretation of cancer progression in images from oncology clinical trials. All the research projects funded by Project Data Sphere are "leveraging the consolidation of data to do something that is not available otherwise," Louv said.

Challenges

Platform Usability

Platforms, such as Project Data Sphere, rely on data providers for quality assurance of the data to be shared. Providers, in turn, rely on the platform to ensure the terms of the data use agreement (DUA) are met, Louv said. With regard to the former, Louv said Project Data Sphere

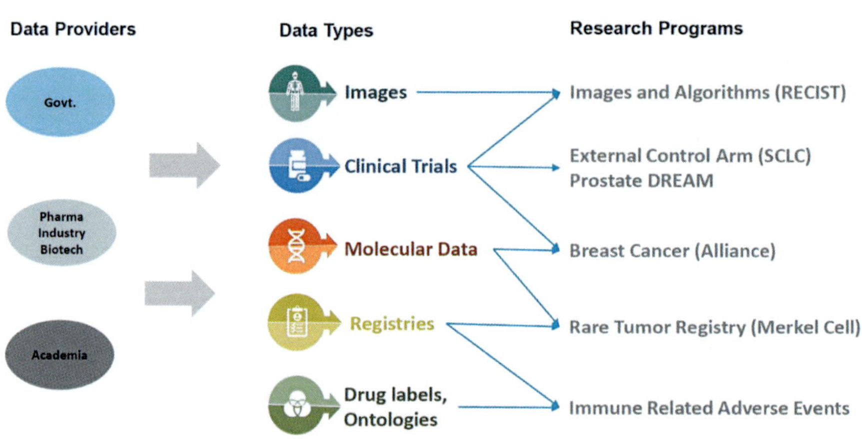

FIGURE 5-2 Project Data Sphere funded data-to-research programs.
NOTE: DREAM = Dialogue for Reverse Engineering Assessments and Methods; RECIST = Response Evaluation Criteria in Solid Tumors; SCLC = small cell lung cancer.
SOURCE: As presented by Bill Louv, November 18, 2019.

assumes that providers will adhere to its recommended standard for sharing data (Clinical Data Interchange Standards Consortium [CDISC]), will properly deidentify data, and that the metadata provided match the data files. A challenge, he said, is that data files "decay" over time as files in the database go unused and those most familiar with the data move on. To address this, Louv said that Project Data Sphere implements a "light-touch dataset acceptance protocol" before including data in the platform. Project Data Sphere also focuses on the usability of metadata, optimizing it for searchability. Louv noted that they have learned from Vivli's work on curation of metadata.

With regard to controlling access to the data, Louv reiterated that Project Data Sphere has an open-sharing model and allows users to download datasets. A challenge for open-access models is that the nature of their openness can be a barrier—causing some data generators to choose not to share on Project Data Sphere. He said, however, that the other data-sharing platforms are also "self-selected groups" and that self-selection of where to share by data providers limits the ability to compare the metrics across platforms.

Data Interoperability

As discussed throughout the workshop, data interoperability across platforms is a key challenge. Currently, Louv said, data users must find ways to work across platforms on their own. To address this, Louv highlighted the need to establish "a federation of data-sharing platforms" that would "establish and maintain standard metadata" at both the platform and the study levels.

Interoperability across data domains is also an ongoing challenge. There are particular challenges for sharing imaging and genomic data, for example. Louv said that data standards and deidentification protocols are "less mature" than those for other types of shared data.

Another challenge is that imaging and genomic data are inherently different from other clinical trial data (e.g., outcomes data) and generally exist in different formats and ontologies. Raw imaging and genomic data are often collected in central specialty laboratories that have different data structures, data stewards (who might have different priorities for data sharing), and data deidentification schemes. Louv explained that it can be difficult to associate the deidentified genomic data with deidentified clinical data, often requiring reidentification, linking, and then deidentification again. As a potential solution, Louv proposed to "limit copying of genomic and imaging data into clinical platforms (and vice versa)," and "enable interoperability with standards for core data, and global patient identifiers."

DISCUSSION

A Searchable Catalog of IPD Available Across Platforms

Participants discussed further Tianjing Li's recommendation for a searchable catalog of IPD that is available across different platforms. Deborah Zarin suggested that ClinicalTrials.gov could potentially serve this function, and she encouraged further discussion on this issue with the registry. Brittany Maguire from the Infectious Diseases Data Observatory (IDDO) pointed out that not all trials of interest with available IPD are registered in ClinicalTrials.gov. There are clinical trials in other registries that can be identified via other databases, such as the WHO ICTRP (mentioned by Tianjing Li above). David Sampson of the American Society of Clinical Oncology shared his perspective as a publisher. He suggested that "data platforms … are analogs of journals" and that the data-sharing community should look to journal publishing for lessons learned about ethics, abstracting and indexing, standards, infrastructure, workflows, and tagging content, for example. He suggested that there is a need to form organizations to support data sharing and to help overcome this lack of coordination. Louv observed that there is still much work to be done on the infrastructure for data sharing, which requires funding, and he expressed hesitancy to form organizations in the absence of a sustainable structure. In response to a question from Hawk, Louv elaborated that Project Data Sphere is a not-for-profit organization that is sustained by its membership structure as well as grants and contracts. Money from funders goes both to the research programs as well as to platform improvements.

A Culture of Data Sharing for Oncology Trials

Coetzee asked whether the fact that Project Data Sphere is focused on a single disease state and indication provides an advantage in creating a sustainable data-sharing platform by essentially creating a supportive community. Louv agreed that the exclusive focus on cancer likely did offer an advantage, although he questioned the ability to scale that advantage in a bigger structure. He described the oncology field as a "tight-knit community" and added that the field is somewhat unique in that "it is reasonable to take more risk to find innovation," and that extends to data sharing. Coetzee suggested that the community aspect creates a culture of accountability with regard to data sharing. Louv agreed, but added that when a company is not willing to share information similar to what other companies have already shared, it is important to have conversations to understand why they are hesitant while others are eager. Ultimately, Louv emphasized, there must be respect for each potential data sharer's situation within his or her organization.

Timely Sharing of Data

Matthew Sydes asked whether the analysis described by Hawk (of the pooled data from six celecoxib trials to amplify safety signals) could have been done sooner, or if the analysis was done at the earliest opportunity. Hawk responded that it was done at the earliest opportunity. Specifically, it was the first time his division at NCI attempted to pool safety data from ongoing, publicly funded trials. He described it as "extremely challenging" because they were not aware of existing models for evaluating safety data from ongoing trials, and they were developing the process as expeditiously as possible as they went along. Although dosing was suspended across all six federally sponsored trials of celecoxib after the initial safety finding, he said it took time to convince the sponsors, trial leaders, and DSMBs for each study of the need to compile the data, to then secure DUAs, and to establish the adjudication process to evaluate an event that was not a primary endpoint.

Avoiding Duplication of Effort

Sydes also raised the issue of avoiding unnecessary duplication of effort in secondary analyses. He noted that he was aware of several other efforts to conduct essentially the same meta-analysis that Tianjing Li's student was attempting. Li acknowledged the difficulty of avoiding duplication of effort and said that groups working on the same or similar topics might collaborate.

Data Quality

Paltoo asked panelists to elaborate on data quality challenges relative to interoperability and usability. Louv reiterated that a key challenge is the "perishability" of clinical trial data. In the time since a study has been archived, the technology and analysis software used have often evolved. For example, when the information in the metadata file does not match the actual trial records, it can be difficult to resolve as study staff with knowledge of the trial have moved on or there are not resources to dedicate to preparing the data for sharing. Louv added that, although more recent studies in newer databases are better suited to sharing with respect to data quality, there are often issues that delay or inhibit sharing, such as intellectual property concerns, a publication plan, or pending regulatory activity.

Another challenge, Tianjing Li said, is the difference in quality, consistency, and harmonization between the data that are currently accessible through data-sharing platforms, and the data one might request from trial investigators at academic institutions, which she described could be "much messier" than the data available for use through the data-sharing platforms. Harmonization is a particular challenge. Data collected using the same instrument or scale might be coded completely differently. As an example, she said that in the data gathered for an IPD meta-analysis, "one trial coded race and ethnicity as two variables and another trial coded it as one variable," which she said eliminated the possibility of conducting subgroup analysis by race/ethnicity. She also raised workforce issues as a challenge, and the importance of having people with the necessary skillsets to use shared data "in a meaningful way."

Hawk emphasized the need to standardize the assessment of behavioral variables and other contextual factors in the conduct of Phase 3 trials, and to consistently assess those variables for trials that might offer the most benefit for data sharing. For example, cancer treatment trials have long focused on the treatment being tested, with limited attention to the broader context in which those treatments are being applied (e.g., concomitant use of tobacco or alcohol). Li added that the development and implementation of core sets of outcomes and common data elements would improve the quality of shared data.

Sonali Kochhar suggested that funding infrastructure development could include the development of basic criteria to facilitate harmonization and data comparability (e.g., core outcomes, core data points to collect for each outcome, basic metadata requirements), and funders could encourage academic and industry trial sponsors to follow these basic criteria.

Tianjing Li said that criteria to consider for outcomes include the name of the outcome (i.e., domain), the preferred measurement instrument, metrics (e.g., relative risk, mean difference from baseline and time point), and time points, for example. Variation in these elements can lead to heterogeneity in treatment effect, and makes meta-analysis very difficult, she said. When a trial cannot be summarized in a meta-analysis, it is difficult to include it in the "totality of the evidence" about the intervention. Li referred participants to the Core Outcome Measures in Effectiveness Trials initiative in the United Kingdom as a model.[5]

Trials for Rare, Neglected, and Emerging Diseases

Maguire said IDDO aggregates data on neglected and poverty-related diseases and emerging infections, and that the clinical datasets they obtain

[5] See http://www.comet-initiative.org (accessed March 2, 2020).

are most often from trials conducted by academia and other institutions, not by industry, and are smaller scale. She raised concern about prioritizing data sharing from large-scale, pivotal Phase 3 clinical trials as trials for neglected diseases would be overlooked. "The totality of evidence should be considered when recognizing the value of IPD," she said. IDDO is also using its disease-focused data platforms to develop a research agenda, which, in turn, facilitates the data-sharing process and the reuse of those data. Maguire said that clinical datasets from neglected disease clinical trials are very heterogeneous, and IDDO is currently curating data to CDISC standards. This is challenging for non-industry trials, but it is feasible, she said. In addition, following the CDISC standard helps to inform prospective data collection by researchers.

Louv said there are similar issues for trials of rare diseases. Few randomized controlled trials exist for rare tumors, for example, and Project Data Sphere is developing rare tumor registries to collect high-quality data.

Data Sharing Impacts the Design and Conduct of Future Trials

Tianjing Li added to the comment by Maguire that the IDDO data-sharing platforms inform their research agendas and that their standardization efforts inform prospective data collection. Li observed that although much of the discussion has been focused on the public health impact of data sharing, data sharing influences the design and conduct of clinical trials (e.g., trials intended for sharing are being designed around a set of core outcomes and common data elements and are appropriately powered statistically). This is a positive outcome of clinical trial data sharing that is difficult to quantify, but that should be acknowledged, Li said.

6

Infrastructure Sustainability

Highlights of Key Points Made by Individual Speakers

- Designing trials with data sharing in mind (e.g., adhering to data standards prospectively) could help to reduce the costs of preparing clinical trial data for sharing. (Humphreys)
- Wellcome Trust funding awards will cover the cost of sharing data, but applicants often do not include a data outputs management plan or a specific cost estimate for curation and sharing in their funding request. (Humphreys)
- Anonymizing every dataset involves significant financial and time investment and might be potentially addressed by anonymizing datasets on a per-request basis. (Kulkarni)
- If shared data are not accessed and used, interest in supporting the infrastructure for data sharing could wane. (Kulkarni)
- There is an increasing number of studies submitted to repositories and a growing data user base without concomitant increases in resources for data stewardship and user support. (Coady)
- A lack of standards for metadata impacts data discovery and usability, especially as a repository expands. (Coady)

The next panel to discuss key challenges to clinical trial data sharing and reuse focused on infrastructure sustainability. Georgina Humphreys of Wellcome Trust discussed challenges associated with the costs of sharing from her perspective as a funder of clinical trials. An industry perspective was provided by Pandurang Kulkarni, chief analytics officer and vice president of Biometrics and Advanced Analytics at Eli Lilly and Company, who discussed the experience of Lilly with sharing data first on its own website, then via ClinicalStudyDataRequest.com (CSDR), and now as a member of Vivli. Sean Coady, program officer in the Division of Cardiovascular Sciences at the National Heart, Lung, and Blood Institute (NHLBI), discussed data-sharing infrastructure sustainability challenges from the perspective of an individual from the National Institutes of Health (NIH) institute. The panel was moderated by Timothy Coetzee.

FUNDER PERSPECTIVE

Georgina Humphreys, Clinical Data Sharing Manager, Wellcome Trust

The Wellcome Trust was established as a global charitable foundation in 1936 through an endowment from Sir Henry Wellcome, Humphreys said. Wellcome is "dedicated to improving health for everyone." Based in the United Kingdom, Wellcome currently spends about £1 billion ($1.3 billion)[1] supporting research every year and, Humphreys said, intends that the outputs of that research "be accessed and used in ways that maximize benefit to health and society." She described Wellcome as "a passionate champion and advocate of open access and data sharing … driven by long-standing policies."

Researcher Challenges

Humphreys shared findings from the Springer Nature survey Practical Challenges for Researchers in Data Sharing. She noted that this was a cross-disciplinary survey of more than 7,700 researchers and was not specific clinical research, but the findings are similar to results from a survey of clinical trial researchers that Wellcome and other funders recently conducted.

Researchers surveyed identified the following concerns about data sharing[2]:

---

[1] Estimated dollar figures at the time of the workshop.

[2] A white paper describing the survey findings is available at https://partnerships.nature.com/wp-content/uploads/2019/08/Whitepaper-Practical-challenges-for-researchers-in-data-sharing.pdf (accessed February 10, 2020).

- "Organizing data in a presentable and useful way."
- "Unsure about copyright and licensing."
- "Not knowing which repository to use."
- "Lack of time to deposit."
- "Costs of sharing data."

Wellcome does, in fact, cover the cost of sharing data, and there is a prompt to include an outputs management plan in the funding application, Humphreys said. However, applicants often do not include an outputs plan or a specific cost estimate for curation and sharing.

Cost/Funding-Associated Challenges

Humphreys discussed some of the cost/funding-associated challenges and concerns in three segments of the data-sharing process: (1) the data management plan, curation, and preparation for sharing; (2) storage and management of sharing; and (3) secondary use (see Figure 6-1).

Data Management Plan, Curation, and Preparation for Sharing

One area of concern is building the skill base needed for developing the data management plan, curating the data, and preparing the data for sharing. One option Humphreys described is to permanently embed data stewards in institutions that sponsor clinical trials to support all of the necessary data-sharing activities at the institution. This would help

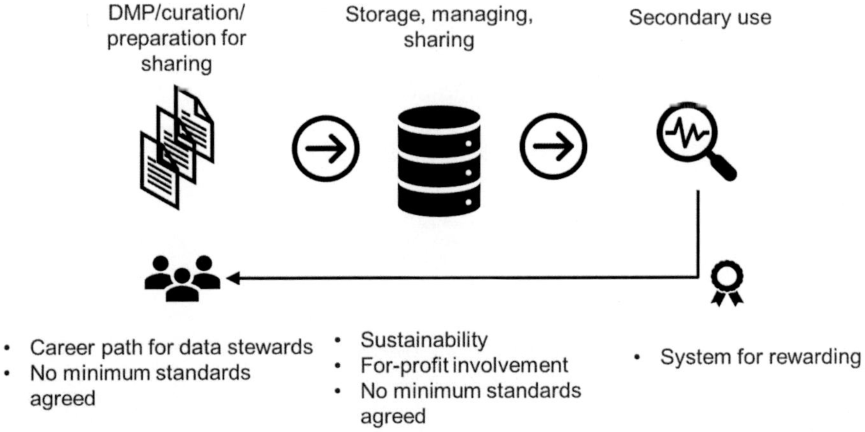

FIGURE 6-1 Costs of sharing.
NOTE: DMP = data management plan.
SOURCE: As presented by Georgina Humphreys, November 18, 2019.

to build institutional skill and expertise in data sharing. She mentioned examples of these efforts already being conducted on a pilot basis in the Netherlands and the Republic of Ireland. One question is how these new positions should be funded. She said Wellcome considers the financial burdens of this endeavor to be an institutional cost that should be supported in the core budget.

Another issue to be addressed is the lack of minimum agreed data standards. Humphreys pointed out that there are standards for pharmaceutical companies that will submit data for product licensure, but there is not yet any agreement on data standards among academic researchers.

Storing Data and Managing Data Sharing

There is a range of options, and costs for storing data and managing the sharing of data, Humphreys said, from a simple deposit to the more involved processes used by platforms that manage requests for data.

Sustainability is a key concern when considering the costs of data storage and management of sharing, Humphreys said. As has been discussed, different funding models are used to support repositories such as grants with fixed timeframes and pay-per-project or membership fee models. A question when addressing sustainability is the expected or needed life span of the repository. She said multiple funding models might need to be used.

Transparency of for-profit involvement in data storage and management is also a concern. Funders need to be aware of the structure of the system they are supporting. Humphreys said funders that receive government or public-based support might find it difficult to justify funding a for-profit model.

As in the first area, the lack of agreed-to standards is also a challenge for data storage and management. Humphreys raised a concern that there are often no minimum standards, even in some of the recommended findable, accessible, interoperable, and reusable (FAIR)-aligned data repositories.[3]

Secondary Use

A concern with secondary use that was raised throughout the workshop was the need to create a system to reward those who contributed data to repositories. Humphreys noted the value of using ORCID IDs[4]

---

[3] See https://fairsharing.org/databases (accessed March 15, 2020) for examples of FAIR-aligned data repositories.

[4] See footnote 3 on p. 12.

and digital object identifiers, which can help funders assess an applicant's track record of data outputs as part of the funding decision. Wellcome asks applicants to submit an output management plan, which she said can include code, data, publications, and samples.

Example: Curation Cost Calculation

To illustrate the cost of data sharing, Humphreys described the work of Catrin Tudur Smith of the University of Liverpool to evaluate the resources needed to share individual participant data (IPD) from a clinical trial. Tudur Smith and a team of experts—including a statistician, a data manager, and a clinical trial manager—prepared IPD from two clinical trials for sharing, documenting the time spent and calculating the cost per team member for their time (Tudur Smith et al., 2017). Humphreys reported that one trial required 50 hours to prepare the datasets for sharing at an estimated cost of more than £3,000 ($3,900), and the other trial required about 40 hours at a cost of about £2,500 ($3,250).[5] She added that this does not take into account the costs of addressing inquiries by data requesters in the future.

Humphreys concluded that designing trials with sharing in mind, including adhering to data standards prospectively, could help to reduce the costs of preparing clinical trial data for sharing.

INDUSTRY PERSPECTIVE

Pandurang Kulkarni, Chief Analytics Officer and Vice President of Biometrics and Advanced Analytics, Eli Lilly and Company

Kulkarni shared how he gained an appreciation for the complexity of clinical trials after moving from academia to industry. Large trials can have thousands of participants, years of follow-up, numerous variables, and large datasets. He said it can be challenging to understand the information associated with a large clinical trial unless one has had experience conducting clinical trials.

As part of its ongoing commitment to transparency, in 2014 Lilly launched a company website for researchers to submit requests for access to Lilly clinical trial data. Later that year, Lilly transitioned data-sharing activities to CSDR, and in 2019 Lilly joined as a member of Vivli. To date, Lilly has spent more than $3 million on infrastructure for analysis and data anonymization, Kulkarni said, and dedicates about three full-time equivalent staff resources per year. Moving the data-sharing process to

[5] Estimated dollar figures at the time of the workshop.

BOX 6-1
Proactive Clinical Trial Data Sharing by Lilly

What Lilly Shares

"Lilly will list Lilly-sponsored interventional clinical studies from approved medicines and indications in the United States (US) and European Union (EU) in the following categories:

- Phase 2, 3, or 4 studies used as part of a regulatory approval submitted to the US FDA [U.S. Food and Drug Administration] on or after 1999.
- Phase 2, 3, or 4 global studies in indications approved in both the US and EU with a first patient visit after 1 January 2007.
- Phase 2, 3, or 4 regional/local studies in indications approved in both the US and EU with a first patient visit after 1 January 2014."

When Lilly Shares

"Studies are listed 6 months after the studied medicine and indication have been approved by regulators in the US and EU and after the primary manuscript describing the results has been accepted for publication, whichever is later."

SOURCES: Kulkarni presentation, November 18, 2019, from https://vivli.org/ourmember/lilly (accessed February 10, 2020).

Vivli has reduced some of the staffing needs and costs, he continued, and Lilly is working to reduce the costs of standardizing and anonymizing the data. He added that, in 2014, FDA implemented requirements for adherence to certain standards for regulatory submissions (e.g., the Clinical Data Interchange Standards Consortium [CDISC] Study Data Tabulation Model [SDTM] and Analysis Data Model [ADaM] standards),[6] which means that Vivli member companies are all submitting data that have been standardized in a similar fashion. The parameters of what Lilly shares proactively are summarized in Box 6-1.

A participant observed that Lilly's $3 million spent on data-sharing activities is likely a very small fraction of the company's overall research budget. Kulkarni agreed but said that the $3 million could have been used to instead support the development of a therapeutic molecule. The company fully supports investing in data sharing, and he clarified that his

[6] Further information on SDTM and ADaM are available in the FDA Data Standards Catalog. See https://www.fda.gov/industry/fda-resources-data-standards/study-data-standards-resources (accessed February 10, 2020).

point was to emphasize the need to use the data resources that are being made available for sharing.

Lilly Data Request Process

The process for accessing Lilly clinical trial data begins when a researcher searches for Lilly studies on the Vivli data-sharing platform and then submits a hypothesis-testing proposal for the studies of interest, Kulkarni said. Lilly ensures that the data are available to share, and Vivli might ask for clarifications on the proposal. The completed proposal is reviewed by the independent review panel (managed by Wellcome Trust), a data use agreement (DUA) is signed, and the data are then made accessible in the secure research environment for the researchers' analyses. John Grecula of The Ohio State University asked about any authorship conditions in the DUA. Kulkarni said Lilly only requires that publications acknowledge the use of data from a Lilly-sponsored clinical trial.

Kulkarni said that Lilly had originally considered anonymizing every dataset created, but, given the significant expense, it decided to wait to see how many requests for data were actually received. The number of requests has been relatively low, and Lilly has decided to anonymize on a per-request basis, he said. He added that automation of the process has decreased the time needed.

More than 350 Lilly clinical trials are now listed on Vivli, Kulkarni said. Since 2014, 78 proposals have been submitted, 40 of which requested Lilly data only and 38 of which requested a combination of Lilly and other sponsors' trial data. Ninety percent of the proposals requested data from oncology or neuroscience trials. Of the 78 proposals, he said that 50 were approved and given access to the requested data. The remainder are still being processed, were withdrawn, or were rejected by the independent review panel (IRP), Kulkarni explained. Of the 50 proposals approved, 12 have resulted in publications.

Commitment to Data Sharing

Lilly is committed to sharing clinical trial data, and Kulkarni said that data sharing "is part of the normal process of conducting clinical trials for Lilly." In addition to listing trials on the Vivli platform, Lilly also participates in Project Data Sphere and the TransCelerate Placebo and Standard of Care Data Sharing initiative.[7] The latter has allowed Lilly to use shared control arm data to inform trial design and, in some cases,

[7] See https://transceleratebiopharmainc.com/initiatives/placebo-standard-of-care (accessed February 10, 2020).

"to replace some part of the placebo arm using data from TransCelerate," Kulkarni said. Lilly also shares data through the disease research foundations working on lupus, Alzheimer's disease, and Duchenne muscular dystrophy. Kulkarni supported the concept of a single data-sharing platform where researchers could access thousands of trials.

In closing, Kulkarni said that Lilly has invested significant time and resources making trial data available for sharing, but secondary use of the data is still very limited. He expressed concern that if shared data are not being accessed and used, interest by data generators in supporting the infrastructure for sharing could wane.

PLATFORM PERSPECTIVE

Sean Coady, Program Officer, Division of Cardiovascular Sciences, National Heart, Lung, and Blood Institute

Coady discussed data-sharing infrastructure sustainability challenges from the perspective of an individual NIH institute. A key aspect of sustainability is an institutional commitment to sharing, Coady said, and NHLBI leadership has been committed to wide sharing of data for more than 30 years. NHLBI's first data-sharing policy was instituted in 1989 by then director Claude Lenfant, who committed to making deidentified data from contract-supported studies available. Although there was then a formal policy in place to enable sharing, few in the research community knew about it, Coady said.

In 1999, protocols to implement the data-sharing policy were developed, and the NHLBI Data Repository was established, Coady continued. The NIH-wide data-sharing policy was released in 2003, requiring grant applicants to include a data-sharing plan with their application.[8] To provide a means for NIH grantees to share their data per the NIH requirement, in 2005 NHLBI expanded the scope of its data repository to include investigator-initiated (i.e., grant-supported) studies in addition to the contract-supported studies already included. In 2009, NHLBI created the Biologic Specimen and Data Repository Information Coordinating Center to facilitate integrated searching of both the data repository and the institute's existing BioRepository.[9] The current NHLBI director, Gary Gibbons, established the Trans-Omics for Precision Medicine program in 2014, facilitating the sharing of more than 150,000 whole genome

---

[8] See https://grants.nih.gov/grants/guide/notice-files/not-od-03-032.html (accessed March 31, 2020).

[9] See https://biolincc.nhlbi.nih.gov/home (accessed February 10, 2020).

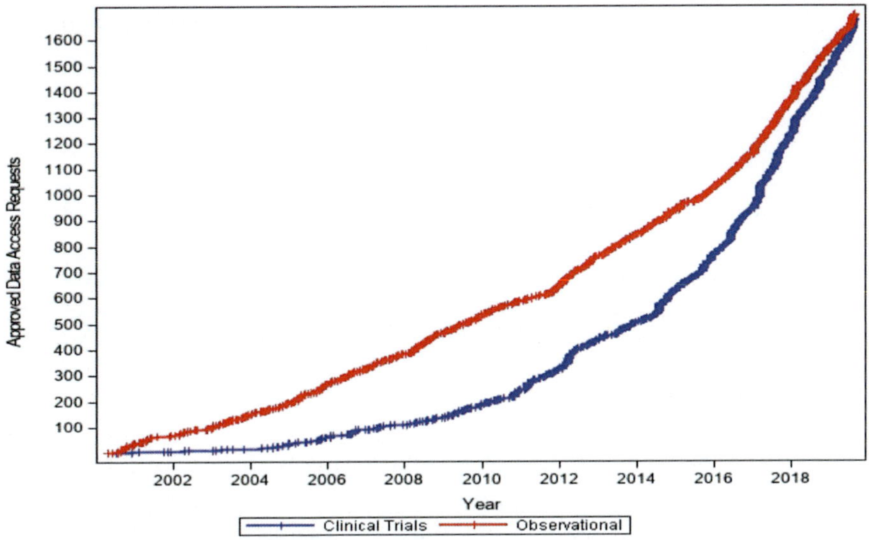

FIGURE 6-2 Increasing demand for access to study data in the National Heart, Lung, and Blood Institute data repository.
SOURCE: As presented by Sean Coady, November 18, 2019.

sequences and other omics data.[10] In 2019, the institute began development of BioData Catalyst, a cloud-based infrastructure for data and tools built on a data commons approach to sharing and data science.[11]

Challenges

Coady highlighted several concerns in the areas of platform usability, resource constraints, and outcome metrics, pointing out that his perspective on the challenges facing platforms is similar to those expressed by other workshop panelists.

Usability and Resource Constraints

Coady showed a graph of the cumulative data access requests for both clinical trial and observational data in the NHLBI registry, which illustrates the increasing rate of demand, especially for clinical trial data (see Figure 6-2).

[10] See https://www.nhlbiwgs.org (accessed February 10, 2020).
[11] See https://www.nhlbidatastage.org (accessed February 10, 2020).

He elaborated on several of the challenges of accommodating this growing user base.

- **Metadata standards.** Coady described the NHLBI data repository as a "come as you are" repository of clinical trials and observational studies and said that the lack of standards for metadata impacts data discovery and usability, especially as the repository expands.
- **Stewardship burden.** NHLBI conducts a review of data that are submitted to the repository, Coady said. Reviewers confirm de-identification and usability factors (e.g., accurate coding, alignment of the metadata with the clinical data). He added the growing number of studies submitted to the repository further constrains resources.
- **Implicit user support.** When investigators access data in the NHLBI repository, it is understood that staff will attempt to answer any questions investigators might have. A concern, Coady said, is that the repository continues to grow, but resources do not grow simultaneously, making it increasingly more difficult to provide the support that is implicitly assumed.

Outcome Metrics

Some of the outcome metrics used to evaluate an institution's investment in a data-sharing platform are relatively simple to assess, such as the number of website visits or the number of data access requests fulfilled. Using the number of publications as a metric can be burdensome, Coady said, as there is often the need to search for them. Other metrics that would be useful to have, but are more difficult to track, include the use of shared NHLBI data for workforce training and the inclusion of shared data in follow-up grant applications.

Coady shared that the NHLBI repository has generated more than 1,100 publications over the past 20 years, about half of which were based on clinical trial data and about half on observational study data.[12] Sixty-eight trials from the repository have led to one or more publications, and investigators who published tended to publish more than once, he said. He added that it took about 5 years before half of the data users published their first paper, which is something for newer registries to keep in mind when looking at metrics.

---

[12] See https://biolincc.nhlbi.nih.gov/publications (accessed March 15, 2020).

DISCUSSION

Priorities

Coetzee prompted participants to identify additional priorities to address sustainability challenges (aside from funding). Coady reiterated that metadata standards would help to accelerate discovery and help to maintain longer-term usability. Kulkarni agreed and said that CDISC metadata standards are used by the pharmaceutical industry, and he suggested that academic researchers also consider using CDISC standards as a base, rather than creating new standards. He also reiterated his support for the concept of a single data-sharing platform to overcome the problem of not being able to combine datasets from different platforms. Humphreys agreed that the lack of standards is a priority item and suggested that there is a need for an internationally recognized body to convene stakeholders and drive the standard-setting process. Amy Nurnberger referred others to the Research Data Alliance, which has convened working groups to consider standards, including metadata standards, for specific fields, including health (although not specific to clinical trials).[13]

Concerns About Using Multiple Platforms

Matthew Sydes observed that Lilly is contributing data to three of the five data-sharing platforms that were discussed, and Wellcome Trust oversees the IRP for two of the five. He asked if different Lilly trials are deposited in different repositories, and which platform a researcher interested in Lilly datasets should use to begin with. From a sustainability perspective, he questioned whether all of these platforms are needed. Humphreys clarified that Lilly transitioned from CSDR to Vivli and is not contributing to both simultaneously. She confirmed that the same Wellcome IRP provides services to CSDR and Vivli, using the same criteria for both. She explained that she serves as the point of contact between the two platforms and ensures that, if researchers submit the same or similar proposal to both, the IRP does not consider it twice. She noted that many of the clinical trials that Wellcome funds are conducted at centers that use their own data access committees, and she said it could be argued that they are not independent. She suggested that a single IRP for multiple platforms could provide consistency across platforms. Kulkarni acknowledged that Lilly is willing to support multiple data transparency activities (including, as mentioned, TransCelerate and Project Data

[13] See https://www.rd-alliance.org (accessed February 10, 2020).

Sphere), but that it is resource intensive, and a single platform would be more sustainable and usable.

Preservation of Data Beyond Platform Life Span

David Sampson from the American Society of Clinical Oncology raised a concern about data preservation if a platform is not sustainable. He noted that there are archives that can preserve the content of journals that cease publication. Kulkarni said that, although he could not comment on the platforms, Lilly and other pharmaceutical companies preserve data per regulatory requirements, and after preservation is no longer mandated, companies archive data so that they can be retrieved if needed (although he noted there might be time and cost involved to retrieve). Data are assets to companies, he said, and they are well preserved. Coady said the NHLBI platform uses accession numbers with versioning so that when older editions of studies are archived, they can be referenced through the accession number. Coetzee observed that, while industry preserves data as an asset, this factor is not a motivation for all data generators. He suggested there might be a need for standardization of preservation, or important datasets could be "lost to history."

Data-Sharing Cost Estimates

Given the different estimates of the costs of data sharing that have been discussed, Jeffrey M. Drazen asked how NIH might calculate allowable data-sharing costs. Humphreys agreed that the numbers discussed are just estimates and are very heterogeneous. She speculated that many of Wellcome's grant applicants do not include an estimated cost for a data outputs plan in their applications because they do not know what that cost would be. Wellcome deliberately does not specify allowable amounts to enable applicants to be flexible in how they propose what is needed for their specific project, she said. Coady said that investigators initiating large clinical trials are encouraged to consider data-sharing costs as part of an overall data management process. Alex Sherman added that, years ago working with the Critical Path Institute, they calculated the costs of the activities needed to merge data from multiple trials in the same disease space to be $25,000 to $30,000.

Costs of Providing IPD to Participants

A workshop participant said that clinical trial participants generally have the right to their own patient-specific data from trials and asked how frequently such requests are made and what the costs of fulfilling the requests are. They suggested that if thousands of participants in a large trial requested their individual data, the costs could be high. Kulkarni responded that the trial sponsor is never in direct contact with participants, and that it would be a trial investigator who receives and fulfills the request from the patient. Sherman said that clinical research organizations routinely deliver trial participant data to each site, and the cost of providing an individual's clinical trial data would be essentially the same as that for other participants at the same site. The challenge in delivering a specific participant's file is that the data provided are only identified by subject ID, he said, and only the site knows each identity.

Data Obsolescence

Drazen asked about the actual use of archived historical datasets, especially when clinical practice has changed over time (e.g., the treatment of heart attacks over the past several decades), and whether there is a time when a dataset is obsolete. Coady cited several older NHLBI clinical trials from which data are still being requested and used to consider various associations (e.g., the Studies of Left Ventricular Dysfunction from the 1990s). He said there are many uses for old data, especially with new statistical methods (e.g., risk factor identification, risk prediction).

7

Challenges and Disincentives for Sharing and Reuse of Data

Highlights of Key Points Made by Individual Speakers

- A challenge for academic clinical research units is meeting data access requests after trial oversight and data access committees disband following completion of a trial. (Sydes)
- Specific training courses could be developed for new researchers requesting data for secondary uses. (Sydes)
- Expanding the knowledge base about the complex biology of disease involves effective partnerships that enable access to both data and expertise. (Daron)
- Elements of effective partnerships and alliances for data sharing include the ability to execute, the ability to learn and grow, and shared value. (Daron)
- Ongoing discussions about the benefits and risks of clinical trial data sharing are primarily about how data sharing might impact researchers and study sponsors, not about what is needed from a participant perspective. (Terry)
- Institutions conducting trials often use issues such as participant privacy or the costs of data sharing as excuses for not sharing. (Terry)

The third panel to consider key challenges to clinical trial data sharing and reuse examined challenges and disincentives. Matthew Sydes, professor of clinical trials and methodology in the Medical Research Council (MRC) Clinical Trials Unit at University College London (UCL), discussed four key challenges to sharing and reuse of data from his perspective as a researcher. Ramin Daron, vice president for data architecture and technology at Takeda Pharmaceuticals, drew from his experience as a sponsor of clinical trials and discussed the importance of effective partnerships to facilitate data sharing and discover new insights. Sharon Terry, president and chief executive officer of Genetic Alliance, shared her perspective as the head of a patient-focused research advocacy organization and the parent of two children with a genetic condition. The panel was moderated by Dina Paltoo.

RESEARCHER PERSPECTIVE

Matthew Sydes, Professor of Clinical Trials and Methodology, Medical Research Council Clinical Trials Unit, University College London

Sydes shared an observation from serving as chair of the Scientific Committee for the International Clinical Trials Methodology Conference (ICTMC) in Brighton, United Kingdom, in 2019. This was a large conference of primarily academic clinical trialists and methodologists, and he said that of 500 abstracts, only 4 (less than 1 percent) were focused on methodological issues of clinical trial data sharing.[1] Sydes then discussed four challenges to sharing and reuse of data from his perspective as a researcher.

Using Data in a Valid Way and Utility of New Knowledge

As a clinical trialist, Sydes said he is working to "maximize the highest quality science to have the greatest societal benefit," both in association with clinical trials and in related research. He highlighted some of the challenges of ensuring that shared trial data are used in a valid way and that the new knowledge generated from data sharing is useful.

Opportunity Costs

There are opportunity costs to be aware of when clinical trialists become engaged in supporting secondary research, he said. As discussed throughout the workshop, it takes effort to create datasets suitable for sharing, including both designing trials from the start with the intent to

[1] ICTMC 2019 meeting abstracts are available at https://trialsjournal.biomedcentral.com/track/pdf/10.1186/s13063-019-3688-6 (accessed February 10, 2020).

share as well as preparing the relevant documentation after trial completion. These activities are costable (i.e., a monetary value can be assessed), he said. However, effort is often expended to support datasets after release. Data users might contact the trial investigators with questions about the data, and this engagement can lead to greater involvement in the secondary research than expected. Supporting these uncostable secondary activities presents an opportunity cost. Secondary research can lead to important findings, but Sydes noted that an issue is the degree to which the MRC (the core funder of the MRC Clinical Trials Unit at UCL) expects these activities to be supporting this work.

Protecting Trial Integrity in Secondary Uses

Sydes emphasized that "trials are analyzed by highly qualified teams" according to pre-specified statistical analysis plans that provide details about planned primary, secondary, and exploratory analyses and that account for the potential for statistical errors associated with multiple testing. Extensive subgroup analysis by trial teams is often criticized as essentially searching the data for findings ("trawling the data"). He said some International Committee of Medical Journal Editors journals exclude subgroup analyses from abstracts, even when they have been detailed in the statistical analysis plan. He added that there are also concerns about the reproducibility of results from some less well-planned studies, which he noted is currently a particular concern in the psychological literature.

Protecting the integrity of the original clinical trial and fostering integrity of secondary analyses are ongoing challenges. To help address this, Sydes offered several suggestions applicable to researchers requesting data for secondary analyses:

- Data requesters could be required to define analyses in advance. Sydes said that guidance for developing statistical analysis plans for clinical trials could inform secondary analysis plans as well (e.g., Gamble et al., 2017).
- Applicant qualifications could be logged.
- An "approved researcher status" could be created to register vetted researchers.
- Users of shared data could be asked to repeat analyses from the original trial to demonstrate that they understand the datasets.
- Specific training courses could be developed for new researchers requesting data for secondary uses. Sydes added that completion of training could be added to one's curriculum vitae and noted on data request applications.

Rationale for Accessing Trial Data

Sydes said it would be interesting to better understand the motivations for accessing shared clinical trial data. His unit has been logging users' intent and has found that many data requesters are planning to conduct individual participant data meta-analysis, while others are seeking linkage to biological samples. Sydes speculated that some of the applicants for data access are not actually interested in individual clinical trials (i.e., comparative data) but are instead seeking "prospectively collected, high-quality data." For example, they might be seeking data estimating event rates in a particular population, and a particular trial is a means to obtain a sample set. He also speculated that if researchers could obtain access to real-world data, such as routinely collected data in the electronic health record (EHR), that might better suit their analysis needs and reduce the applications for access to clinical trial data. He acknowledged that there are challenges specific to accessing and sharing routinely collected data that are beyond the scope of the workshop, but noted that there are parallels with some of the challenges discussed thus far for sharing of clinical trial data.

Oversight Process for Access to Shared Data

Another challenge for sharing data is the oversight process for clinical trials. Sydes explained that in the clinical trial unit where he researches, oversight is a three-part system: a trial-specific Trial Steering Committee (TSC) that is assembled for each trial involving independent members; an Independent Data Monitoring Committee (or referred to by some as a Data and Safety Monitoring Board, Data Safety Monitoring Committee, or Data Monitoring and Ethics Committee); and a Trial Management Group (responsible for day-to-day trial activities).

Requests for data span the length of a trial and beyond (see Figure 7-1). Sydes said a few requests might be received during trial recruitment or early in the trial before the primary analysis (e.g., event rate data from the control arm). Most requests are received after the primary analysis is completed, and requests can continue for some time after the trial is completed. The TSC usually fulfills the data access role, Sydes said, but they and the other oversight committees generally disband after the trial, if not earlier. This leaves a void in reviewing data access requests and results in trial investigators filling requests. He said they are now working toward establishing a unit-wide Data Access Committee, with the intention of ultimately contributing trials to an external data repository and thereby reducing the trial team's input into how the trial data are used for secondary research in the longer term. Sydes observed that there is limited discussion of when the process of reviewing data access requests should move from internal to external.

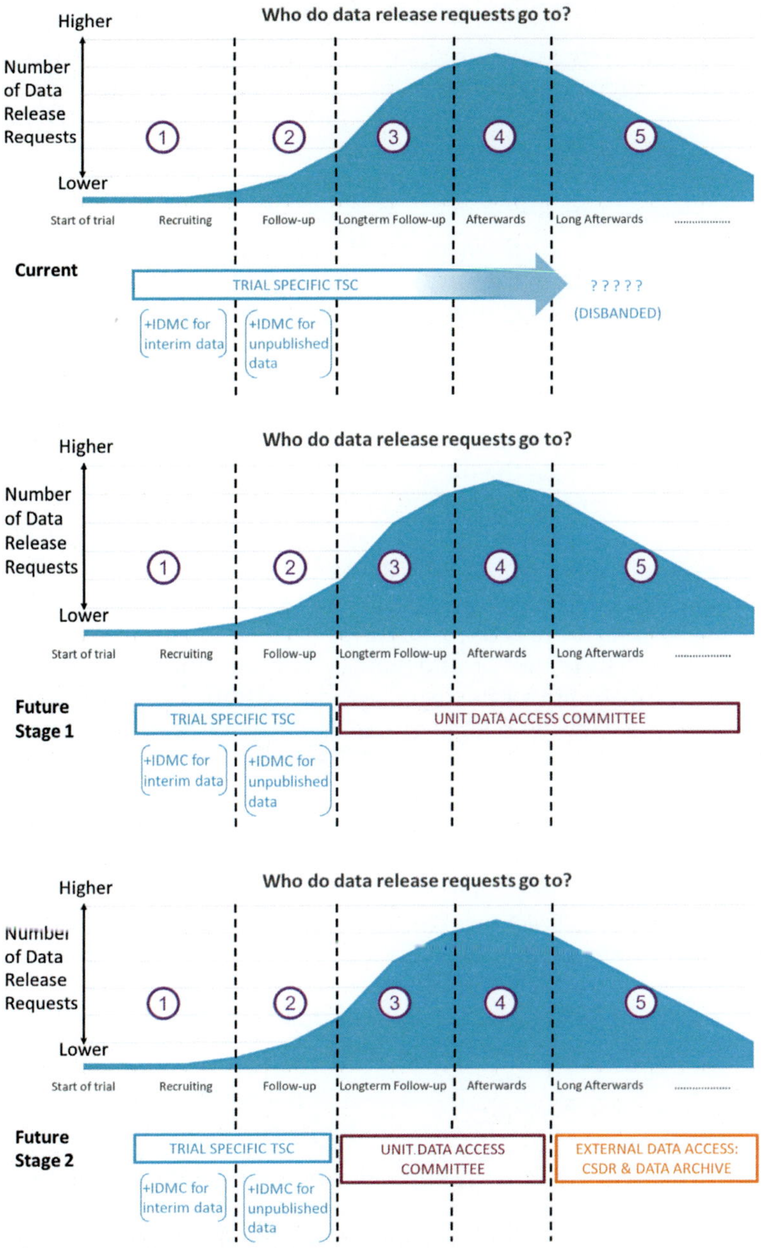

FIGURE 7-1 Oversight and timing of data release requests.
NOTE: CSDR = ClinicalStudyDataRequest.com; IDMC = Independent Data Monitoring Committee; TSC = Trial Steering Committee.
SOURCE: As presented by Matthew Sydes, November 18, 2019.

Recognition of Data Generators

The last challenge discussed by Sydes was addressing the need for recognition and reward of researchers involved in generating and sharing clinical trial data. Using an example of three people in the entertainment industry, all with the last name of Jones (a well-known American actress, a UK actor, and a makeup artist), he illustrated the value of a database that links individuals to their body of work. Using the Internet Movie Database (known colloquially as IMDb), one can find information about individuals (e.g., all roles a person in the industry has filled across projects, regardless of whether they had top billing as a star or worked behind the scenes) and about projects (e.g., every person credited for a film and their role).

Sydes proposed that a similar type of database is needed for those who contribute to clinical trials (Sydes and Ashby, 2017). Recognizing contributors with authorship goes against strict journal guidelines for authorship and is not practical given the thousands of people whose work contributes to a clinical trial. For example, there are pharmacists, radiologic technologists, data managers, and numerous others who help to facilitate clinical trials and produce the dataset, who are not generally recognized. To illustrate, he described a large-platform trial that has been ongoing for several years that has thus far produced 11 editorials and 30 papers.[2] Collectively about 150 people have been authors on those publications; however, 3,500 additional staff are currently listed on delegation logs, and about 100 others are former staff who have or had roles on the team.

Perhaps an "IMDb for clinical trials" could use digital object identifiers, ORCID IDs,[3] or other unique identifiers to link researchers and datasets they have contributed to, and enable better recognition of these contributions, Sydes suggested. Such recognition could help to alleviate some of the concerns about data sharing. He noted that there are logistical issues to consider, such as whether one digital object identifier would be issued per trial, or one for each version that is uploaded to a data-sharing platform, or whether there are differences between academia and industry with regard to recognition. He added that new models for recognition would need buy-in from promotion committees and publishers.

Other Challenges

Other challenges briefly mentioned by Sydes included anonymization (e.g., how and when to properly anonymize/de-link datasets), and how to return results of trials to participants, especially results of secondary analyses (e.g., who has responsibility, who funds).

---

[2] See https://clinicaltrials.gov/ct2/show/NCT00268476 (accessed March 30, 2020).

[3] See footnote 3 on p. 12.

SPONSOR PERSPECTIVE

Ramin Daron, Vice President, Data Architecture and Technology, Takeda Pharmaceuticals

Daron acknowledged the workshop discussions thus far on the challenges associated with data quality, incentives, costs, and infrastructure, and focused his remarks on several other issues, including the importance of effective partnerships. Expanding the knowledge base about the complex biology of disease "takes the work of many," Daron said, and involves partnerships that enable access to both data and expertise. Drawing from his experience as a sponsor of clinical trials, Daron listed three elements of effective partnerships and alliances:

1. **Ability to execute.** This includes elements such as standardization, normalization, and stabilization to increase efficiency.
2. **Ability to learn and grow.** Daron observed that adaptability and willingness to try new approaches can seem at odds with standardization and other elements of efficient execution, and it is important to develop an understanding of what stakeholder needs are (e.g., open access, restricted access).
3. **Shared value.** Alignment of goals and objectives better enables partners to resolve issues and overcome challenges to move forward.

Case Example: Overcoming Internal Data-Sharing Challenges

To illustrate the importance of partnerships, Daron describe an example of overcoming data-sharing challenges internally within Takeda. Historically, only certain teams have had access to the data for particular clinical trials, he said. Researchers often find themselves at odds, with some on the "defense"—striving to maintain the integrity of the trial and the validity of the interpretations—and others on the "offense"—eager to identify novel insights and new approaches.

The company decided to try to move the mentality about internal data sharing from "why do you want access?" to "why can't you have access?" Daron said there was a need to "build trust and transparency between the different functions and the teams" and to define shared goals for the use of the data. In reviewing the organizational and functional aspects of the company and assessing the internal competencies and capabilities, it was found that simply sharing data more broadly by creating data libraries would be insufficient. There was also a need for libraries of analytics and utility.

Takeda has worked to develop these libraries and the internal capabilities for data interoperability and reuse (e.g., data standards, analytics). He said this has allowed the company to maintain the integrity of its clinical trials while also facilitating the identification of errors before database lock. Better internal sharing of trial data has also enabled new insights and enhanced the efficiency of translational research.

Case Example: Learning from Failures

Another example of the value of data sharing is the potential to gain new insights from failed clinical trials that did not meet predefined outcomes, Daron said. Examining data from failed trials for anomalies and aberrations can, for example, find subpopulations who responded exceptionally well to an investigational treatment even though the overall trial results were not statistically significant. These types of findings can help to elucidate the biology of the disease or the mechanisms of action of the product. As a result, the company has begun "deep phenotyping" of participants with anomalous results to better understand the reasons behind them. Daron said Takeda is also reaching out to other pharmaceutical companies and academic researchers to potentially share data and increase the statistical power for these small populations.

PATIENT PERSPECTIVE

Sharon Terry, President and Chief Executive Officer, Genetic Alliance

Terry shared her perspective as the head of Genetic Alliance, a patient-focused research advocacy organization and as the parent of two (now adult) children with a genetic condition. She is also the founder of a research advocacy organization and biospecimen bank for that condition. Terry shared that when she established the disease foundation 25 years ago, she insisted on data sharing by the researchers studying that condition. (In a process she described as herding cats by moving the food, data sharing was a condition of access to biobank samples.) Terry said her interest is in making data sharing easier. This will require an "industry shift," and she suggested looking to other industries that have transformed themselves for lessons.

The Missing Perspective

Terry described how the perspective of the patient as both generator and user of data is still not present in research. Institutions and organizations are the decision makers, and questions are still asked and answered from the perspective of researchers. "Every single one of us is a patient," Terry said, and researchers need to bring that perspective to their work.

Ongoing discussions about value versus the risk/cost of clinical trial data sharing are primarily about the benefit/risk for researchers and study sponsors, she observed, and not about what is needed from a participant perspective. She suggested that institutions conducting trials often use issues such as participant privacy or the costs of data sharing as excuses for not sharing. Instead of transparency being the norm, terms such as "risk of audit" suggest a fear of transparency, she said.

Although secondary use is discussed primarily from the perspective of researchers, Terry noted several examples in which the public is using shared data for research. Shared data are commonly used by disease advocacy groups, as well as by interested individuals and affinity groups such as Pennsylvanians concerned about the health impacts of fracking or parents concerned about soccer-related head injuries. Terry cited the success of the Systolic Blood Pressure Intervention Trial Data Analysis Challenge and called for greater sharing of data with the public for their use, and better engagement of the public in the citizen science–type of activities that are common in other fields.

Case Example: Platform for Engaging Everyone Responsibly

Terry described Genetic Alliance's Platform for Engaging Everyone Responsibly (PEER) as an example of a public data-sharing initiative.[4] PEER, launched 10 years ago, is a cross-disease database in which individuals enter and control the sharing of their own health-related data with advocacy organization–sponsored registries. PEER currently has approximately 50,000 individual users representing about 100 diseases, with participation from 25 disease advocacy organizations. PEER recently partnered with LunaPBC, a public benefit corporation, for platform support.

Despite initial concerns about sustained participation, Terry said that PEER participants have remained interested. She credited this interest to the ongoing engagement that is at the core of the initiative. PEER participants answer questions asked by validated patient-reported outcome instruments and can upload EHR and genomic data, all of which remain in full control with regard to sharing. PEER participants can also receive shares of the genomic data platform, LunaDNA, for contributing their genomic and other information. They can decline the shares, hold the shares, or donate them. Terry explained that Luna received approval

[4] See http://www.geneticalliance.org/programs/biotrust/peer (accessed February 10, 2020).

from the U.S. Securities and Exchange Commission for this, and is the only company granting shares in exchange for data as a currency. Terry acknowledged the concerns expressed by many in the field that commerce should not be part of data sharing. She countered that commerce is already involved in data sharing, and there is financial benefit for everyone except the individuals whose data are being shared.

Terry announced that PEER will soon be conducting a clinical trial in the platform in collaboration with a company. PEER participants will be messaged anonymously through the platform and can choose to be part of the trial. She explained that the sponsor will add data to each participant record in real time, which means there is no lag time in the return of data to trial participants, and also facilitates use of data as they are generated. PEER also has a "virtual data analysis sandbox," which she explained allows researchers to conduct analyses on data in the platform, as well as securely upload their own analysis tools and proprietary datasets for use, and to share findings to the PEER participants' records. Terry said this sandbox approach reduces some of the infrastructure burden for academic investigators, and also allows for reproduction of analyses and longitudinal follow-up. She added that PEER has a system for credentialing researchers and for data use agreements.

A key challenge is that there has been minimal interest in supporting a "people-run entity" that is not associated with a company or an academic institution, Terry said. Support has come from a variety of sources, including, she said, "cake sales and car washes." Support from a company for the upcoming clinical trial is an important step, she said, and she added that she looked forward to the outcome of the study.

DISCUSSION

Paltoo asked panelists about data-sharing challenges that might be encountered in association with special or unique populations. As an example, Terry said that concerns about data sharing have been expressed by Native American populations and by patients with sickle cell disease. A feature of PEER allows advocacy communities to create a default data-sharing setting for participants to use. She said members can choose to use it or not, but that "most people will follow their gatekeeper or their key opinion leader" regarding sharing. She emphasized that one size does not fit all. Each individual has preferences, and the platform allows each community to set parameters. Many communities tend to want to share data only with researchers who are aligned with the community, and whom the community already knows and trusts, Terry said. However, after having a positive experience with sharing their data, many do agree to expand their circle.

Sydes raised the issue that consent for pediatric populations is given by parents or guardians, and technical re-consent is required when the child reaches legal age so the status could change. Sydes also reiterated the point from an earlier discussion that if data are not shared from the entire trial cohort, that can lead to bias in any subsequent analyses, including meta-analyses (i.e., the patients shared do not fully represent the trial data).

8

Finding Value in Sharing Clinical Trial Data: Overcoming Usability and Sustainability Challenges

Highlights of Key Points Made by Individual Speakers

- The goal of clinical research synthesis is to "maximize the relevance and utility of clinical research to clinical practice." (Helfand)
- There is a need to prioritize the sharing of data that clinicians and patients need to use, and reward data reuse for validation and to answer questions that will help clinicians and patients make informed decisions. (Helfand)
- Motivations for data sharing include fulfilling a responsibility to trial participants to reap the most benefit from their data; fulfilling the conditions of funding awards; and recognition as a data source in a publication or opportunities for a co-authorship. (Bertagnolli)
- Data sharing is enabled by planning to share from the start, using standard data formats, and access to resources, including data platforms and people and expertise. (Bertagnolli)
- Data standards should be platform independent and should be addressed in the planning stages of studies, and existing standards should be leveraged rather than creating more. (Kush)
- Technical barriers to data sharing can be overcome with standards and harmonized common data models; however, cultural, political, and legal barriers can persist. (Kush)

In this session, panelists explored opportunities and potential solutions for overcoming the technical and sustainability challenges discussed throughout the workshop. Mark Helfand, professor of medicine, medical informatics, and clinical epidemiology at Oregon Health & Science University, shared his perspective as user of shared data for research synthesis. Monica Bertagnolli, professor of surgery at the Harvard Medical School, provided the perspective of an institution that generates and shares data. Rebecca Kush, chief scientific officer at Elligo Health Research, discussed next steps from a platform perspective. The panel was moderated by Ida Sim, professor of medicine at the University of California, San Francisco, School of Medicine.

Sim provided a brief review of the many components of data sharing that were discussed thus far in the workshop relative to the components of the data-sharing environment (see Figure 8-1).

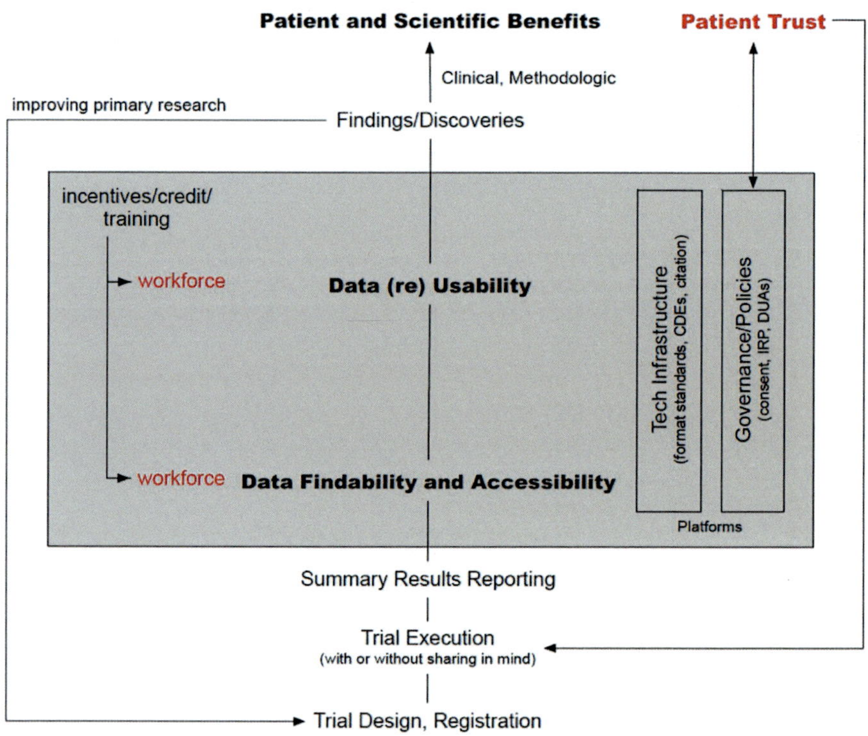

FIGURE 8-1 Representation of the data-sharing environment.
NOTE: CDE = common data element; DUA = data use agreement; IRP = independent review panel.
SOURCE: As presented by Ida Sim, November 19, 2019.

The findable, accessible, interoperable, and reusable principles[1] state that data should be findable, accessible, interoperable, and reusable. One suggestion to address barriers to findability and accessibility, Sim said, was to create a single portal to search for individual participant data across platforms (ClinicalTrials.gov and the World Health Organization International Clinical Trials Registry Platform were both mentioned as models).

Some of the barriers to data reusability have been addressed by the use of data-sharing platforms, which Sim said incorporate technical infrastructure, governance, and policies. Suggestions discussed that would aid usability included standards for both data and metadata (Clinical Data Interchange Standards Consortium [CDISC] was mentioned as an example), and the need for an infrastructure to link an individual's ORCID ID[2] to the digital object identifiers for their contributions.

With regard to governance, it was discussed that the patient voice needs to be at the center of the process. Engaging research participants in decisions about how their data will be shared and used fosters trust in the biomedical research enterprise, Sim said. Maintaining patient trust is essential because without participants, there can be no clinical trials.

Workshop participants also discussed the need for common data request functionality across platforms, and there were suggestions to combine the platforms. In this regard, Sim pointed out that Vivli bridges multiple platforms, and users can request datasets from other platforms (e.g., Johnson & Johnson, the National Heart, Lung, and Blood Institute's Biologic Specimen and Data Repository Information Coordinating Center[3] Project Data Sphere), which can be collected into a secure environment in Vivli for analysis.

With regard to workforce, discussion took place about training, incentives, and ensuring that those who generate and share data receive credit. Developing a career path for data stewards was also suggested.

Data sharing generates new findings and discoveries. One discussion was that these are not only clinical but also methodologic, Sim said, and reuse of data benefits patients and contributes to the scientific knowledge base. The topic of metrics was discussed throughout the workshop, and it was emphasized that there is a need for metrics beyond the number of publications.

These findings and discoveries are not the endpoint, Sim continued, but they feed back and inform the next round of primary research (e.g., trial design, methodology). She noted that improving the process of science is a key benefit of data sharing, and metrics are needed to better understand

[1] See footnote 3 on p. 64.
[2] See footnote 3 on p. 12.
[3] See p. 68 for more information.

the value added. Another point of discussion was that, when data sharing is expected, trials are designed up front with data sharing in mind. One suggestion was to institute auditing of a subset of trials, with the premise being that the risk of audit could inspire uniform data husbandry.

DATA USER PERSPECTIVE

Mark Helfand, Professor of Medicine, Medical Informatics, and Clinical Epidemiology, Oregon Health & Science University

Helfand focused his remarks on overcoming data-sharing challenges as they relate to research synthesis—specifically, systematic review and meta-analysis. Technical issues raised by speakers throughout the workshop included IPD availability and the lack of any centralized, searchable catalog of IPD; insufficient data standardization; and inability to merge data. In addition, Helfand said that "users can't learn everything," elaborating that, for researchers whose primary background is in systematic review and meta-analysis, navigating original clinical trial data can be challenging.

The goal of clinical research synthesis is to "maximize the relevance and utility of clinical research to clinical practice," Helfand explained. Clinicians have difficulty applying clinical study findings in journal articles to practice. Reuse of data for research synthesis can pool results from different studies of an intervention, evaluate an outcome across interventions, and importantly, assess the impact of the way that studies were designed, conducted, and analyzed on the results. Helfand elaborated on several areas for attention from his perspective as a data user.

Mistrust

Helfand observed that there is mistrust of secondary data users, which he suggested stems from the culture of clinical trial science (not from concerns about the data users themselves). In essence, trialists are being asked to trust a data analyst who is not associated with the study to evaluate their work (product, idea, surgical procedure, etc.). He said that activism by patients and clinicians is needed to change this culture. Patients who participate in clinical trials and clinicians who need to apply trial findings to practice should demand that researchers make the best use of participant data.

Data Needs

The depth of metadata needed for systematic review and meta-analysis can be different from that needed for other uses, Helfand said.

Systematic reviewers can find themselves working with trialists to refer back to the raw information from ascertainment, case report forms, and clinical notes to find the necessary metadata. This is generally beyond what platforms can address at this time, Helfand said.

Helfand also raised the issue of using shared data for replication of studies, voicing his disappointment in platforms' experiences so far. Some reported zero data requests expressing intent to replicate studies. However, others reported that all their study replication data requests resulted in perfect replication results. He speculated that the platform process might not be ideal for that type of "forensic" assessment of trials, or that perhaps platforms might be filtering out users interested in replication studies.

Data Sharing and Analysis

Helfand agreed with comments by several other speakers that "systematic reviewers, meta-analysts, and other reusers should have trial experience." He elaborated that trialists use practical and subjective judgment in interpreting data, which data analysts with minimal trial experience tend to label as bias. Analysts without trial experience also tend to rediscover things that are generally already known by trialists. He recommended that the training pathway for data analysts include trial experience.

Helfand also agreed with the suggestions made regarding prioritizing which clinical trial data to share. He continued that the data that clinicians and patients need to use should be prioritized. He added that data reuse for validation and answering questions that help clinicians and patients make informed decisions should be rewarded.

DATA GENERATOR/SHARER PERSPECTIVE

Monica Bertagnolli, Professor of Surgery, Harvard Medical School

Bertagnolli spoke from her perspective as the chair of the Alliance for Clinical Trials in Oncology.[4] A successful clinical trial, she said, "answers important questions, achieves timely accrual of appropriately representative patients, addresses disparities, generates high-quality data, and creates resources for future use," which include data and biospecimens.

Alliance has long been committed to data sharing as a fundamental goal, Bertagnolli said. Alliance has been a member of the National Cancer Institute's (NCI's) National Clinical Trials Network (NCTN) since its establishment in 1955, and was involved in the first multi-institutional

---

[4] See https://www.allianceforclinicaltrialsinoncology.org/main (accessed February 10, 2020).

cancer clinical trial, called "Protocol #1," Bertagnolli said.[5] She added that the protocol was 17 pages long, and four carbon copies were made. In 2007, Alliance began a major commitment to data sharing when the Adjuvant Colon Cancer End Points (ACCENT) Group was established. Researchers in the ACCENT Group agreed that data from their individual trials would be shared and pooled. For perspective on data volume, she said that, in 2010, Alliance had 61 actively enrolling clinical trials when the Alliance Statistics and Data Center was relocated from Duke University to the Mayo Clinic. Although electronic data capture was being used, there were seven semi-truck loads of paper data spanning 1955 to 2010 that had to be moved. The NCTN adopted a network-wide electronic data management system in 2011 for use by all NCTN groups, which Bertagnolli described as "a huge advance." In 2015, the NCI launched its own platform, the NCTN/NCI Community Oncology Research Program (NCORP) Data Archive.

Alliance Contributions to Data Sharing

Alliance currently contributes data to the NCTN/NCORP Data Archive (all studies published on or after January 1, 2015). Studies that were completed before the NCTN/NCORP launch were contributed first to Project Data Sphere and later to Vivli. Biospecimens linked to Alliance clinical trials are contributed to NCTN Navigator, and genomic data are contributed to the database of Genotypes and Phenotypes. All other data requests are handled by Alliance, and Bertagnolli noted that Alliance receives many requests for legacy data.

Bertagnolli summarized Alliance's contributions to data sharing for 2015 through late 2019 as follows:

- NCTN Data Archive: 38 publication datasets from 33 unique trials.
- Project Data Sphere: 22 publication datasets of legacy data from 20 unique trials.
- NCTN Navigator: 40 unique trials covering more than 23,000 patients and 355,000 specimens, 15 requests completed (providing specimens with links to clinical data).
- National Center for Biotechnology Information database of Genotypes and Phenotypes: 5 institutional review board–approved data transfers for 4 unique trials.

[5] Alliance in its current form is the merger of the American College of Surgeons Oncology Group, the Cancer and Leukemia Group B, and the North Central Cancer Treatment Group. NCTN was formerly known as the NCI Clinical Trials Cooperative Group Program.

- Alliance (legacy data): 143 datasets shared with 100 external collaborators and 43 Alliance member groups.

Bertagnolli added that from January through October 2019, Alliance received 28 requests for legacy data (15 have been fulfilled thus far). Requests received are reviewed by the Alliance Statistics and Data Management Center (SDMC), which she explained is also responsible for new study design, data quality monitoring, results analysis and manuscript preparation, and Data and Safety Monitoring Board and funding and agency reports for Alliance's clinical research program. "A research group will always … saturate the capabilities of its statistics and data center," Bertagnolli said. SDMC must prioritize, she said, and processing secondary data use requests can take lower priority in an active clinical research program.

Motivations for Sharing

Alliance is motivated to share data for a variety of reasons. Data sharing is, and always has been, a core value of Alliance. Bertagnolli said that Alliance has a "responsibility to clinical trials participants to share data in ways that bring the most benefit to society." Data sharing is also frequently a condition of funding awards, she said, and awards can include support for data-sharing activities. Other motivations are receiving recognition as the source of data in publications, and opportunities for co-authorship on papers when Alliance participates in the study.

Elements of Success

According to Bertagnolli, Alliance data sharing is enabled by three key elements:

1. **Planning.** Data sharing is planned from the beginning and is specified in contracts and agreements as well as participant consent forms. The intent is to share the data widely to reap the most benefit.
2. **Data standards.** The merging of the cooperative group leads to the use of one standard system, which she described as a major improvement. Alliance is also working toward expanding the use of standard data formats to cancer control and EHR-based data.
3. **Resources.** One valuable resource is the availability of data-sharing platforms for use by Alliance. Another important resource is the Alliance Data Sharing Working Group, which comprises Alliance volunteers and staff and is funded by the Alliance Foundation. Bertagnolli acknowledged three Alliance Data Sharing Champions,

Selina Chow of the University of Chicago, who chairs the data-sharing working group; Sumithra Mandrekar of the Mayo Clinic, who is the group statistician; and Mark Watson of Washington University, who is the Alliance biorepository director. She also acknowledged the many researchers at Alliance member institutions who make oncology clinical research a priority.

PLATFORM PERSPECTIVE

Rebecca Kush, Chief Scientific Officer, Elligo Health Research

Kush discussed data usability challenges from a platform perspective. She shared a Venn diagram, originally created in 1997, and said it represented an approach for automating electronic health records extraction of clinical research case report form data in order to optimize clinical research. Standards were clearly needed and, she said, they needed to be independent of any specific platform or technology. At that time, initial standards had been developed by HL7[6] and CDISC. In 2004, the NCI, the U.S. Food and Drug Administration (FDA), HL7, and CDISC came together to develop the Biomedical Research Integrated Domain Group (BRIDG) model to bridge clinical research and health care, enhancing data interoperability.[7] Kush said that the BRIDG model is now a global standard, which has been approved through HL7, CDISC, and the International Standards Organization. In 2010, through the Healthcare Information Technology Standards Panel/American National Standards Institute, an interoperability specification (IS #158) was developed for using EHRs for research, identifying standards from HL7 and CDISC and integration profiles from Integrating the Healthcare Enterprise to support this use case. In 2016, FDA and the Japanese Pharmaceuticals and Medical Devices Agency began requiring that data in regulatory filings be submitted in a CDISC standard format, which Kush noted that other countries have now endorsed.[8] Most recently, HL7 has released its Fast Healthcare Interoperability Resources (FHIR), and the National Institutes of Health is evaluating how this standard might be used by its grantees. Kush referred participants to several recent publications that support the value of using standards for data sharing (see Kush, 2014; Kush and Goldman, 2014; Ohmann et al., 2017; Varnai et al., 2014).

---

[6] For more information on HL7, see http://www.hl7.org (accessed February 10, 2020).

[7] See https://bridgmodel.nci.nih.gov (accessed February 10, 2020).

[8] See https://www.fda.gov/industry/fda-resources-data-standards/study-data-standards-resources (accessed February 10, 2020).

Common Data Model Harmonization

Four organizations or networks, Observational Health Data Sciences and Informatics, Informatics for Integrating Biology with the Bedside, the FDA Sentinel Initiative, and the National Patient-Centered Clinical Research Network (PCORNet), currently use four different data models, Kush said, which increases the burden of researchers sharing data to participate in multiple research networks. In addition, she said there has been a proliferation of common data elements, some of which are not necessarily standards, and can potentially leave data gaps in databases, including inadequate metadata. To address the challenge of low interoperability among networks, FDA has worked on a project with other federal agencies, and with funding from the Patient-Centered Outcomes Research Institute trust fund, to harmonize these four common data models. Because the BRIDG model is broad and robust and is a global standard, it was decided to map the different common data models to the BRIDG model. Terminologies were also mapped and harmonized across these data models.

Elligo Health Research was contracted to identify data partners who would run queries for a pharmacovigilance use case, and thus test the goal of making it easier for participants using the four different data models to participate in research and data sharing by leveraging the products of the common data model harmonization initiative. Kush reported that it was interesting to find that the barriers encountered during the use testing were not as much technical as they were legal, cultural, and political. A second phase of the project will leverage HL7 FHIR.

Summary

In closing, Kush summarized some of the lessons learned and key messages regarding data usability challenges:

- "The technical ability to share meaningful data should be platform-independent, and data standards enable this," Kush said.
- Standards can create efficiencies in research and in data sharing, she added, and should be addressed up front in the planning stages of studies.
- To be most effective, Kush continued, standards and data models need to be broadly adopted and should include metadata.
- "Researchers should leverage existing robust/global standards and data models before creating new ones," she said.
- Technical barriers to data sharing can be overcome with standards and harmonized common data models; however, cultural, political, and legal barriers can persist.

DISCUSSION

What Data to Share

Participants continued the discussion of what data should be shared. Amy Nurnberger advocated that all trials should be shared because the expectation that data will be shared promotes good data management. Also, as discussed, sharing trial data "honors the time and the investment of the participant." Sharing all trial data would also help to reduce duplication and increase efficiency. Helfand said that "all trials" would need to be defined. For example, is there a need to share data from very small trials with no clinical outcomes, or from Phase 1 pharmacokinetic trials? His perspective was that the definition needs to be broader than just Phase 3 trials and beyond. He said, for example, that dose-finding studies would be relevant to share. He explained that his intention is not to restrict sharing but to "set a target for starting, get the data processes right … and eventually expand it to all trials." Bertagnolli said the oncology clinical trial groups are continually funded and supported data centers that conduct many trials, and that all of the publication datasets likely are shared via platforms. However, not all data collected are included in the publication dataset, and groups such as Alliance are needed to facilitate sharing of other data, such as case report forms that include all of the captured data elements. Sim raised the issue of who should make the decisions about the scope of trials to share. Helfand said that as platforms continue to evolve, they will need continued input. The pressing decisions, he said, are not about whether all data from every trial should be shared but, rather, what should be shared for a particular trial. He added, for example, that limiting sharing to publication datasets would not fulfill his analysis interests. Bertagnolli reiterated the value of sharing case report forms.

Frank Rockhold recalled the discussions during the development of ClinicalStudyDataRequest.com (CSDR) regarding which trials to include and said that "the easy decision is all." Although the concept of prioritizing Phase 3 trials is logical, it can be difficult to define what that would include. For example, he said, some Phase 2 trials enroll 1,000 participants. Furthermore, it seems clear that a 15,000-participant outcomes-based cardiovascular disease trial of public health importance should be shared, he added, while there is likely to be little interest by other researchers in a food-effect study of yet another beta blocker. Yet, he said, there would likely be a lot of overlap between Phase 2 and Phase 3 studies. He reiterated his philosophy that trials should be conducted with the expectation that data might be shared. The expectation of future data sharing drives better data husbandry and reproducibility.

Sim agreed that all studies should practice good data husbandry with the expectation of sharing, but added that taking this approach does not mean that all trials need to fully prepare their data for sharing that might not occur. Some activities are time and resource intensive and could be done if and when data are requested (e.g., anonymization). Sim suggested that a useful task might be to define what dataset preparation should be done "in anticipation of a potential request."

Tim Feeney raised the issue of sharing analysis and code along with trial results. He speculated that some requests for data might be simply to check the accuracy of the analysis. In this regard, he noted that there is now a trend toward posting code on GitHub so that others can review the code for errors. Kush mentioned the Mobilizing Computable Biomedical Knowledge initiative,[9] as well as a call for papers describing "computable knowledge" by the journal *Learning Health Systems*.[10]

Replication of Studies

Following up on Helfand's remarks on replication studies, Joseph Ross clarified that there has been only one study using data from the Yale University Open Data Access (YODA) Project for the specific purpose of replicating a particular trial, and there were some discrepancies between the primary report and the secondary analysis. He added that the secondary data users worked with the clinical team regarding issues of replication, which he said provided a better understanding of the metadata needed to replicate the analyses (Gay et al., 2017).

Ross said that replication is one purpose of data-sharing platforms, and he recalled the inability to replicate studies associated with the Merck Vioxx trials due to, he said, changes in the case report forms. He described a current analysis of the impact of data sharing on assessing the cardiovascular risk associated with the diabetes drug Avandia. Using data shared in CSDR, he identified a signal of cardiovascular risk that was not apparent from analyzing the summary data in the clinical study reports. He emphasized that the main purpose of a data-sharing platform should be to improve the overall understanding of the products tested in the trials and to enable other avenues of research (i.e., not detecting misconduct or other challenges).

Helfand noted that the publication of the Merck Vioxx Gastrointestinal Outcomes Research trial did mention cardiovascular effects in the discus-

[9] See https://mobilizecbk.med.umich.edu (accessed February 10, 2020).

[10] See https://onlinelibrary.wiley.com/pb-assets/assets/23796146/Computable%20Knowledge%20Paper%20Author%20Instructions-1561647093960.pdf?campaign=dartwol%7C5124726649 (accessed February 10, 2020).

sion, and FDA was aware of the concerns from the data in the regulatory submission. In writing a report for Medicaid, Helfand used the statistical and clinical summaries available on the FDA website, which he said included detailed analysis of the cardiovascular effects. He suggested that the regulatory role in data analysis is being overlooked, and added that he questioned the justification for replication analyses "validating what FDA has already discovered." He observed that promotional materials and journal articles often do not fully reflect the data that are already in the public domain.

Rockhold supported the need for reproducibility and replicability of studies but cautioned that, just because another group cannot replicate the original study, it does not mean they are correct and the original research is flawed. Helfand agreed and added that there can also be different interpretations of data. As was observed in the Systolic Blood Pressure Intervention Trial, for example, many opinions were expressed about the relevance of the findings to clinical practice. The medical establishment is familiar with disagreement, and he cited the American College of Physicians and American College of Cardiology guidelines, which have interpreted studies differently. Helfand and Rockhold both said that different findings by a reanalysis is an opportunity to learn and do not necessarily mean one study or the other is wrong.

Engagement of Original Researchers

Matthew Sydes asked Bertagnolli to elaborate on the ways in which data sharing can lead to co-authorship on publications. For example, to what extent might collaboration with original researchers happen when data are shared via a repository versus a trials group such as Alliance? "When is it important to seek the engagement of the original researchers?" he asked, and what role do independent review panels (IRPs) play in facilitating or hindering collaboration? Bertagnolli said the study statistician is the original study team member most frequently engaged as a collaborator for the data requests received by Alliance. Data requests are reviewed by the Alliance working group, and also by the original study statistician, who can best address questions about the feasibility of the proposal. The statistician is also usually engaged in the secondary analysis. She added that she was not aware of a collaboration that had resulted from the sharing of a legacy trial through one of the platforms, but she acknowledged that Alliance does not track data that have been contributed to the platforms. Sydes asked about when a trial should be contributed to a data-sharing platform (versus sharing via a trials group website), and whether the original trial team should continue to be engaged in review of data access requests submitted to platforms.

He noted concern that a platform IRP cannot be expected to have the same depth of expertise in any given study as the original research team would. Bertagnolli clarified that all of Alliance's publication datasets are submitted to a platform, unless prohibited by legacy third party agreements. Alliance researchers engage if asked, she said, but all requests for access to publication datasets are handled by the platform.

Sydes asked whether there is information about the extent to which contact with original study teams is made through a platform versus directly. Sim said that Vivli data requesters know who the data contributor is, and data contributors are informed that their data have been requested and by whom, but Vivli leaves it to the parties to contact each other if desired. Platforms cannot require collaboration, she said, but they could potentially take measures to make the process easier. She noted that Vivli does not yet formally track collaborations but said that this question was an interesting one. Helfand shared that, for one of the early YODA Project studies, Yale served as an intermediary among groups; he added that he did not know the extent to which this intermediary role happens now. Helfand also noted that there are other potential intermediaries, such as funders; he also raised a concern that original investigators might seek to have more control than perhaps they should (e.g., over what is emphasized, how results are disseminated). These issues are difficult to address in a DUA, he said, and he emphasized the need for intermediaries but added that there is not clear guidance available on negotiating such collaborations.

Managing Workload

Bertagnolli reiterated that the vast workload of a statistics and data center will persist, as will resource constraints. She agreed with others that the solution is to plan for sharing from the outset so that there is no need to go back and prepare data for sharing at the end. Sim asked if that planning takes into account the statisticians' time to work with data requesters (e.g., salary support). Bertagnolli responded that Alliance does fund the working group that reviews the requests. Jeffrey M. Drazen asked about handling the increased workload when a secondary analysis identifies an inconsistency or error in a shared dataset. Bertagnolli said they have not had this experience yet. Sherman shared that his group has experienced this, and they "dropped everything" to address it. They also then announced the issue and resolution so others who might have used those data could reevaluate.

Common Data Models

Ross said that aligning with common data models will be especially important as clinical trials increasingly rely on data from health systems.

Joanne Waldstreicher mentioned that companies are working together to develop master protocols, which she said ensures that sponsors are collecting the same endpoints and outcomes, and are using the same definitions and other parameters. Sponsors are also developing platform trials in several disease areas, which she said helps to reduce the number of participants needed in control groups and allows for "more meaningful comparisons on both efficacy and safety across different treatments."

Choice of Data Standards

Alex Sherman observed that shared trial data will likely be in CDISC format as that is the format required by FDA for regulatory submission, but said that CDISC is not intuitive to many researchers. He asked Kush if other formats might be better for sharing. Kush responded that "there is no right or wrong when it comes to standards." It is a matter of building consensus and all parties coming to agreement about which standards to use, then adopting these broadly and using them as the foundation for extensions such as therapeutic area–specific standards.

9

Looking Forward: Incentivizing Data Sharing and Reuse

Highlights of Key Points Made by Individual Speakers

- To be of value, data should be shared in a way that works for data users; otherwise, all the effort that goes into sharing will be wasted. (Roberts)
- The value of shared data for secondary use could increase through adherence to standards; clarity in trial sponsors' data-sharing policies; therapeutic area data pooling by sponsors; and the development of findable, accessible, interoperable, and reusable multi-stakeholder platforms. (Roberts)
- Individual participant data (IPD) meta-analysis is "the highest form of value that one can derive from a randomized trial." (Baigent)
- New, rigorous research is needed that classifies and evaluates the range of different outputs from data sharing, including outputs that are of societal value. (Baigent)
- Data professionals—including data stewards, curators, librarians, archivists, and others—are part of the infrastructure that needs to be built up and better leveraged for clinical trial data sharing. (Nurnberger)
- The use of persistent unique identifiers for datasets can enable the tracking of citations as an output of trial registration. (Nurnberger)

- Open sharing of clinical trial IPD can lead to direct impacts on patient care. (Humphreys)
- More input is needed from researchers in low- and middle-income countries because they face different challenges and have developed different solutions from those of researchers in high-resource settings. (Humphreys)

In the final session of the workshop, panelists considered steps needed to incentivize and promote data sharing and reuse. Liz Roberts, senior director and global public policy lead at UCB Biosciences, discussed how trial sponsors could make shared data more useful to secondary data users. Colin Baigent, deputy director of the Clinical Trial Services Unit and Epidemiological Studies Unit (CTSU) at Oxford University, provided examples of how individual participant data (IPD) meta-analysis can lead to new and important findings that impact patient care. Amy Nurnberger, program head of data management service at the Massachusetts Institute of Technology (MIT), discussed the roles and relationships of institutions and other clinical research stakeholders in sharing trial data, and the value of engaging libraries in data management activities. Georgina Humphreys, clinical data sharing manager at Wellcome Trust, discussed Wellcome's broad approach to maximizing the value of research data and how open sharing of clinical trial IPD can lead to direct impacts on patient care. The session was moderated by Roberts. Closing remarks were then provided by Joanne Waldstreicher and Jeffrey M. Drazen.

SPONSOR PERSPECTIVE

Liz Roberts, Senior Director and Global Public Policy Lead, UCB Biosciences

Roberts drew on her experience in industry, primarily as a data generator, but with some experience as a data user.[1]

Value Proposition for Data Sharing

The concept of value-based transparency means sharing information that adds value, not sharing for the sake of sharing. In this regard, Roberts said there is little value, per se, in pharmaceutical clinical trial sponsors listing their trials for IPD sharing. A website with a long list of trials does

[1] Roberts stated that these views are her personal views, and not necessarily those of her company or any other company.

not add value in itself. To be of value, researchers need to be able to find the right trials for their proposals. She said this requires data generators and users working together toward their shared goal "to find new scientific insights and advance human health care."

Advancing human health care is one of the main value-based motivations for pharmaceutical companies to share data, Roberts said. As has been noted by other speakers, she said there is an increasing recognition of the role of trial participants and that responsible sharing of data is a sign of respect for their contribution. She emphasized that sharing must be done responsibly, and there are legal frameworks (e.g., data sharing and use agreements), secure sharing environments, and other structures to help ensure this.

To be of value, Roberts said, data must be shared in a way that works for data users. Otherwise, she said, all the effort that goes into sharing is wasted. Data generators and data users need to work together to find solutions to the challenges of data sharing, Roberts emphasized. To illustrate, she said there have been many cases where her company has approved a data request, signed the data use agreement, and uploaded the anonymized IPD that was requested by a research team, only to find that they never returned to access the data in the system. She said these missed opportunities suggest that the right value proposition has not yet been found.

Challenges and Solutions

A paradigm shift is needed in the clinical research environment, Roberts said, and she offered several solutions for further consideration.

- **Standards.** The need for standards has been discussed by many panelists. Roberts said that volumes of documentation accompany IPD. Although companies share the same information (e.g., clinical study reports, case report forms, protocols, statistical analysis plans, etc.), it is likely in different formats, which is a challenge for researchers to navigate.
- **Clarity in data-sharing policies.** Policies for which data are shared and when vary across clinical trial sponsors, and it can be challenging for researchers to know when data might be available for analysis. Roberts observed, for example, that some will share Phase 1 trial data, while others are less comfortable in doing so. Data might be made available to share after publication of the primary manuscript, or after regulatory approval in one or more countries. Greater clarity is needed in company policies regarding the availability of trial information, she said.

- **Therapeutic area data pooling.** Roberts suggested that, for a particular therapeutic area, companies could agree to use the same data standards, use the same trusted third party to anonymize data using the same algorithm, and pool their datasets, making them available to researchers. She acknowledged that there could be obstacles to overcome, but that this approach could help to reduce the challenges researchers face when navigating the different formats used by different companies.
- **Findable, accessible, interoperable, and reusable (FAIR)[2] multi-stakeholder platforms.** Another potential solution is the development of a multi-stakeholder platform to make it more transparent for researchers to find the data they need for analyses. The goal is to maximize the clinical utility of the data being shared, Roberts said, while ensuring that participant privacy is protected. There is a lot of information being shared on platforms and company websites, she said, and the challenge is for the research community to be able find it. Trial datasets that are shared need to be FAIR, and she noted the value of digital object identifiers.

Key Players

Roberts highlighted three key functions in the data-sharing process that add value. The role of the independent review panel (IRP) in assessing the scientific merit of data requests submitted to platforms is an important element of the data-sharing process, she said. The sponsor should not be the judge for what research should be allowed. Funders are essential for their support of clinical trial data generation outside of industry research and development, she continued, and there are valuable data being shared by academic researchers. Finally, the International Committee of Medical Journal Editors (ICMJE) policies that address prospective trial registration, data-sharing statements in manuscripts, and the inclusion of a data-sharing plan in trial registration have enabled sponsors to plan up front and to better coordinate the roles within the company that are involved in the process of data sharing.

Looking Forward

A host of incremental improvements can be made to enhance clinical trial data sharing, such as reducing the cycle times for completing data-sharing requests, Roberts said. But she believed it is time to focus on a paradigm shift in the environment. She emphasized the need to "start

[2] See footnote 3 on p. 64.

with the end in mind" by picturing the future and designing trials accordingly, rather than attempting to retrofit solutions.

RESEARCHER PERSPECTIVE

Colin Baigent, Deputy Director,
Clinical Trial Service Unit and Epidemiological Studies Unit,
Oxford University

Baigent discussed extracting value from shared clinical trial data to enhance patient care from his perspective as an IPD meta-analyst and as a data sharer through his role as director of the Medical Research Council (MRC) Population Health Research Unit.

Societal Value of Sharing Clinical Trial Data

A variety of different analyses can be conducted using randomized controlled trial data, and Baigent mapped them according to their relative societal value (see Figure 9-1). The predefined primary outcomes of a randomized controlled trial are analyzed by the principal investigators and the research team. Subsidiary analyses are also done (e.g., for secondary outcomes), most often by those involved in the conduct of the trial, and analysis of exploratory outcomes can be used to inform new research. Baigent pointed out that these three types of analyses "respect the randomized structure" and should therefore not be impacted by bias. Non-randomized analyses that ignore the treatment allocation might also be done, but these are subject to bias, especially index event bias. As shown in Figure 9-1, Baigent said that exploratory and non-randomized analyses are generally of lower value to society. At the other end of the scale is IPD meta-analysis, which he argued is "the highest form of value that one can derive from [re-use of] a randomized trial." He added that a value assessment of the different types of analyses of randomized controlled trial data is needed.

The Value of IPD Meta-Analysis of Shared Data

To illustrate the ways in which IPD meta-analysis can lead to new and important findings, Baigent described an analysis of data by the Cholesterol Treatment Trialists' (CTT) Collaboration.[3] CTT was established in 1994 to conduct systematic analyses of IPD from statin trials, which, at the time, were individually of insufficient size to study mortality out-

[3] See https://www.cttcollaboration.org (accessed February 10, 2020).

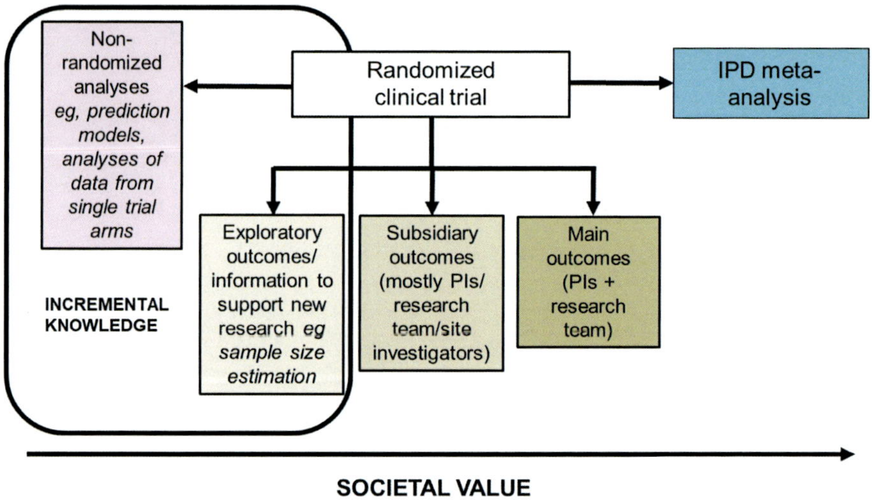

FIGURE 9-1 Learning from shared clinical trial data.
NOTE: IPD = individual participant data; PI = principal investigator.
SOURCE: As presented by Colin Baigent, November 19, 2019.

comes. There were no data-sharing platforms at the time, he noted, and collaborators were requested to share a very specific, standardized dataset from their trial (baseline data; vascular events; cancer; all-cause mortality; demographics; and lipid profiles at baseline, 1 year, and at the final visit). CTT has assembled data from 28 statin trials of 175,000 participants, and its meta-analyses have produced 10 major publications that have collectively been cited more than 10,000 times. This long-term database is maintained by the CTSU at Oxford, and Baigent emphasized the need to preserve such databases independent of the potential uncertainties of data-sharing platforms. He then discussed several of the ways that IPD meta-analysis of shared trial data can provide increased value.

Effects on Particular Outcomes

IPD meta-analysis allows for analysis of intervention effects on individual components of an outcome. Baigent explained that individual trials generally record a limited number of outcomes, and findings are often reported relative to a composite outcome (e.g., heart attack, stroke, death). The first CTT meta-analysis in 2005 studies the effect of lowering low-density lipoprotein (LDL) cholesterol on the incidence of major vascular events. Data were assembled on 13,000 events that occurred in the treatment and control groups of 14 statin trials (data are numbers of events, not numbers of patients with events). Baigent showed that the effects of lowering LDL on each of the different types of vascular events (coronary events, stroke, and coronary revascularization procedures) were similar for a given reduction in LDL cholesterol. However, when the individual components of these outcomes were evaluated, it became clear that the number of hemorrhagic strokes was not reduced. These findings are not apparent when considering the trials individually. In addition, IPD meta-analysis allows for reporting of relative risk reduction per/mmol reduction in LDL cholesterol (which accounts for dose variation across trials).

Timing of Treatment Effects

IPD meta-analysis allows for understanding the timing of a particular effect. Baigent described a different analysis that showed the effect of lowering LDL cholesterol on major vascular events over time. The data suggest that the effect during the first year of statin treatment is half of what it is in later years. This finding is also not apparent from the individual trial data, he said. This finding from the meta-analysis is important for the design and interpretation of trials of LDL-lowering therapies. For example, he said the trials of PCSK9 inhibitors were about 2 years long, and the effects were less than expected. By analyzing shared data on statin therapy, it was able to be determined that this finding was related to the short duration of the PCSK9 trials.

Definition of Whom to Treat

IPD meta-analysis can be used to determine whom to treat. Most trials are powered so that they determine whether to use a treatment for a particular condition. The example Baigent described showed the protective effects of lowering LDL cholesterol in individuals with different baseline LDL cholesterol levels. The IPD meta-analysis found that participants still experienced the protective benefit of lowering their LDL cholesterol levels with statin treatments regardless of their levels at the start of the trial. This is of value, he said, because people can have low LDL cholesterol levels and still be at high risk for a cardiac event. The meta-analysis shows that lowering LDL cholesterol is still beneficial for high-risk patients who do not have high LDL levels.

Unanswered Questions in Need of New Trials

IPD meta-analyses can help to define the research agenda. Baigent described data from a presentation given originally to the U.S. Food and Drug Administration that showed the effects of statins according to baseline renal function. The meta-analysis found that data from individuals with a low glomerular filtration rate were limited. Identifying this gap led to a randomized controlled trial of 9,500 patients, which found that reducing LDL cholesterol is effective in reducing vascular events in this particular subpopulation, members of which, he said, were not being prescribed statins at that time.

Patient Safety

CTT is currently conducting an IPD meta-analysis of all adverse events recorded in the trials in its database. Baigent said that misinformation about the adverse effects of statins is spreading, and the analysis will look for evidence of any association of statin use with increased risk for a range of adverse events.[4] A challenge, he said, is that the original request for trial data was for a defined standard dataset, as discussed above. For this meta-analysis, CTT had to ask for a new dataset from the original trials and then merge the new and old datasets. Clarifying the risk of adverse events will be of high value to patients on statin therapy, he said.

Baigent added that, for a variety of reasons, it has not been possible to leverage all of the data-sharing platforms to gather and maintain the necessary data for this analysis (e.g., the need to maintain the data locally). In this regard, he emphasized the importance of data structures that can support IPD meta-analysis in the long term. A viable approach, he continued, is to enter data use agreements (DUAs) with trial sponsors to share their data, as has been done in the past.

Potential Next Steps

These examples demonstrate how IPD meta-analysis is a high-value use of shared randomized controlled trial data and "can provide enormously important data to help manage patients," Baigent concluded. However, data-sharing platforms are not ideally suited for IPD meta-analysis when multiple sponsors are involved. In particular, data need to be maintained locally for flexibility in analysis (e.g., multi-variate modeling).

Various platform metrics have been discussed throughout the meeting (e.g., numbers of data requests, datasets provided, publications). What is needed, Baigent said, is new, rigorous research that classifies and evaluates the range of different outputs from data sharing, including outputs that are of societal value.

---

[4] See https://www.sciencedirect.com/science/article/pii/S0002870316000326 (accessed April 1, 2020).

Baigent concurred with the remarks by other panelists that the focus should change from making all trials available for sharing to making the most informative data available (e.g., from pivotal studies) and encouraging their reuse. He agreed that attention should be on collecting and maintaining data in a form suitable for sharing, but not necessarily routinely depositing it somewhere.

INSTITUTIONAL PERSPECTIVE

Amy Nurnberger, Program Head of Data Management Services, Massachusetts Institute of Technology

Nurnberger, Program Health of Data Management Services at MIT Libraries, discussed stakeholder roles in sharing trial data and the value of engaging libraries in data management activities. She adapted the five laws of library science by S. R. Ranganathan to data science: "Information, or data, [are] for use, … for every person there is information they are looking to use, for every piece of information there is a potential user, … save the time of the user, … the library is a growing organism."

Realizing the Value of Data Sharing

Nurnberger asserted that the value of data sharing is worth the cost but said there is "infrastructure debt" to be addressed to fully realize that value. First, as has been discussed, Nurnberger said that clinical trial data need to be FAIR. She pointed out that the FAIR principles, as outlined, refer to machine actionability of data (i.e., computational capacity to interact with data). This capacity is still evolving, and with it, the potential of FAIR data. As an example of building on the promise of FAIR data, she mentioned the Personal Health Train being developed by the Dutch Techcentre for Life Sciences.[5]

Another issue is the need for a data-sharing incentive structure and the ability to award credit. Nurnberger suggested looking to other disciplines for technologies and lessons. She also referred participants to the Make Data Count project.[6] She called on participants to advocate for and use persistent unique identifiers for their datasets, which enable tracking of citations as an output of trial registration.

A persistent concern is the limited number of publications stemming from shared data. Nurnberger recommended reaching out to researchers who have not followed through on their data request to find out why. In

[5] See https://www.dtls.nl/fair-data/personal-health-train (accessed February 10, 2020).

[6] See https://makedatacount.org (accessed February 10, 2020).

other disciplines, she said, concerns about being able to trust the data or whether the data will be fit for a researcher's intended use are among the reasons that shared data are not employed. She mentioned the Data Nutrition Project as an example of how the quality of a dataset might be communicated to interested researchers.[7]

Clinical investigators and researchers are not trained in data management or making data FAIR, Nurnberger continued. Data professionals—including data stewards, curators, librarians, archivists, and others—are part of the infrastructure that needs to be built up and better leveraged for clinical trial data sharing. She mentioned the EDISON project of the European Commission, which is working to build the data profession.[8]

Responsibility for Data Sharing

Nurnberger diagrammed the complex "constellation of responsibilities" for data sharing. She focused her comments on the roles and relationships of institutions, funders, and researchers—but first acknowledged some of the other key contributors that have promoted a cultural shift toward sharing and transparency. These include publishers (especially the ICMJE policies that address data sharing); societies and associations (including the National Academies' Roundtable on Aligning Incentives for Open Science); and industry efforts to share data through platform initiatives (e.g., Yale University Open Data Access Project, Supporting Open Access for Researchers, Vivli, CSDR, and others).

Institutions

Institutions are the operational frameworks in which research is conducted, Nurnberger said. Institutions have roles and responsibilities associated with the following:

- Fulfillment of grant terms
- Promotion and tenure
- Legal concerns, such as compliance with data privacy and data-sharing regulations, legal interoperability of data, and balancing legal risk and academic responsibilities in DUA
- Institutional review boards and ethical participant consent
- The research environment (e.g., facilities, technology, infrastructure, grant support systems, libraries)

[7] See https://datanutrition.org (accessed February 10, 2020).
[8] See https://cordis.europa.eu/project/id/675419 (accessed February 10, 2020).

With regard to the research environment, Nurnberger noted that the European Commission has recommended that 5 percent of research expenditure be allocated to research data management. In the United States, she said, libraries have shifted personnel and services to support the research environment. Libraries have expertise in data management, metadata, and privacy, for example, and she encouraged participants from academia to engage their libraries.

Funders

Funders have a broad scope of operation and influence. They establish requirements and structures. Nurnberger suggested that an important role for funders is following up with grantees. Requirements encourage change, she said, but they can be ineffective without follow-up.

Researchers

Researchers have many responsibilities, such as grant term fulfillment, and are essentially responsible for "adherence to everything," Nurnberger said. She noted that investigators often spend time on data management activities for their projects, which should be handled by data managers, and she called on funders and institutions to support data managers for research teams. She also called on researchers to make their support for technology and library initiatives known to their institutional administration.

Researchers also have responsibility for the research culture, she said. They shape the culture through their participation in research, publishing, peer review, service on editorial boards, and roles as program officers in funding agencies. That culture is perpetuated in the promotion and tenure processes and is passed on to students. She encouraged researchers to devote course time to "considering the implications of data management and sharing to instill a respect for the practice and its practitioners." Researchers will not necessarily handle the data management, but there needs to be an awareness that it must be done, she said.

All Stakeholders

All stakeholders are responsible for working together to create a workable research environment, Nurnberger said. Shared responsibilities include developing platforms and standards (building, supporting, and using them), and addressing workforce issues.

Participants and Providers

At the center of the constellation are participants and providers who have a responsibility to be educated and conscientious, and "to remind us who we are responsible to," Nurnberger said.

Be FAIR and CARE

As discussed above, FAIR is focused on machine interactions. Nurnberger described the CARE Principles for Indigenous Data Governance, developed by the indigenous data sovereignty community, which include Collective benefit, Authority to control, Responsibility, and Ethics.[9] Nurnberger said these principles, which recognize that people have a role and responsibility in good data practices, are also relevant to clinical trial research and should be considered when addressing issues of data incentives, policies, standards, and governance.[10] "Having the practices, platforms, and policies for good data management, or husbandry, in place to make FAIR data sharing feasible also means that they are there to support legal requirements of [data protection regulations] and moral imperatives of CARE," she concluded.

FUNDER PERSPECTIVE

Georgina Humphreys, Clinical Data Sharing Manager, Wellcome Trust

One of the key impacts of unavailable data is the inability to reproduce the results of published studies. Humphreys summarized that more than half of researchers could not reproduce their own experimental results, and more than 70 percent could not reproduce the work of other researchers.[11] In addition, pharmaceutical companies report not being able to replicate more than 75 percent of the conclusions in the peer-reviewed literature, which she said impacts translation of findings to practice and ultimately affects patient care. As a funder of clinical science, she expressed particular concern about the impact of irreproducibility on patient care, and she discussed Wellcome's approach to maximizing the value of research data.

---

[9] See https://www.gida-global.org/care (accessed February 10, 2020).

[10] Nurnberger stated that her adaptation of the CARE Principles to clinical trial data sharing was done with the permission of the indigenous data sovereignty community.

[11] See https://www.nature.com/news/1-500-scientists-lift-the-lid-on-reproducibility-1.19970 (accessed March 30, 2020).

Open Data Sharing for Direct Impact on Patient Care

One suggested solution to the problem of irreproducibility is to make the data more available, she said. Wellcome Trust has an open-access data policy, and Humphreys said there is emerging evidence across disciplines suggesting more frequent citations of research articles that are linked to open data.

As an example of the impact of open data sharing, Humphreys described the work of the WorldWide Antimalarial Resistance Network (WWARN), where she noted she worked before joining Wellcome. WWARN was founded in 2009 to collate prepublication data from clinical trials of antimalarial drugs for the primary purpose of mapping and tracking drug resistance. The intent was to use this information to influence decisions on resource allocation to better address emerging drug resistance. The challenge, Humphreys said, was that researchers were not willing to share their data, especially prior to publication. To encourage sharing, WWARN created collaborative study groups for researchers to share and analyze IPD. Contributing researchers participated in the secondary analysis process and were authors on many publications. She added that any analyses containing prepublication data would be embargoed until the data contributor had published their work. This approach led to publications with more than 100 authors, she acknowledged, but it demonstrated the potential of precompetitive sharing of data to directly impact patient care.

Humphreys described a specific example in which IPD from more than 7,000 patients across 26 studies of the antimalarial drug, dihydroartemisinin-piperaquine, were pooled for meta-analysis.[12] Over 3 years, a team of five to six people collated, curated, and analyzed the data and found that many younger children were being underdosed (at levels below the World Health Organization [WHO]-recommended therapeutic range), and that the treatment was ineffective. As a result of this study and subsequent modeling studies, WHO updated their malaria treatment guidelines—which, she said, had a direct impact on the treatment of children in malaria-endemic countries.

Maximizing the Value of Research Data

Data sharing is "the right thing to do," Humphreys said, and many of the reasons why were discussed throughout the workshop. However, one single activity will not overcome the challenges of sharing clinical trial

[12] See https://www.wwarn.org/working-together/study-groups/dp-dose-impact-study-group (accessed February 10, 2020).

data, and she said that Wellcome is taking a broad approach to maximizing the value of research data, including the following activities:

- Implementing the Wellcome outputs management policy[13]
- Ensuring that Wellcome research outputs are FAIR (e.g., through the Wellcome Open Research publishing platform and a pilot program with Springer Nature)[14]
- Enabling open research through support of activities that promote a sharing culture and facilitate sharing (e.g., support for National Academies activities; IRP secretariat for Vivli and CSDR; signatory on the Declaration on Research Assessment)
- Awarding funding specifically for innovation in open research

Funder Reflections

As one of the funders of this workshop, Humphreys reflected on the themes and lessons she took away from presentations and discussions.

- More input is needed from researchers in low- and middle-income countries, Humphreys noted, because these researchers face different challenges and have developed different solutions compared with researchers in high-resource settings.
- More input is needed from the data generators' institutions, said Humphreys. Secondary data users discussed the challenges of DUAs and other legal hurdles to successful data requests, and Humphreys suggested that institutions are not always included in discussions of these issues.
- Humphreys added that shared data are not being leveraged effectively for secondary analyses. Pharmaceutical companies and others have invested in systems and platforms for data sharing, but the number of requests to use these data is much lower than anticipated, Humphreys observed. In addition, data requesters frequently "drop out" and do not access the data after receiving approval, or do not complete and publish their proposed studies.
- The costs of conducting secondary analyses remain high, and data harmonization is a challenge, Humphreys summarized. One approach to addressing these issues that was discussed was increas-

[13] See https://wellcome.ac.uk/funding/guidance/data-software-materials-management-and-sharing-policy (accessed February 10, 2020).

[14] See https://wellcomeopenresearch.org/for-authors/data-guidelines (accessed February 10, 2020) and https://www.springernature.com/gp/campaign/Wellcome-RDS-Pilot, respectively (accessed February 10, 2020).

ing the use of standards in prospective data collection, Humphreys recalled. This endeavor will take time, she said, and she cautioned against "enforcing sharing" in a way that leads to the availability of datasets that are of no value for secondary use.

- Bring people together, Humphreys advised, around purpose-driven data sharing and use. As shown in the examples of WWARN and Project Data Sphere, research programs can drive data sharing, Humphreys said; involve those who will use the results (e.g., policy makers, ministries of health).
- Including the voice of the patient in deciding the use of their data is essential, Humphreys reiterated; honor their role as the true sources of the data.
- Learn from the clinical trial registry experience, concluded Humphreys, with regard to driving information sharing forward and creating a paradigm shift.

DISCUSSION

Access to IPD for Meta-Analyses via Platform or Directly

Waldstreicher shared that many research proposals do not require maintaining data locally and can be performed within a secure platform environment. She clarified that, for IPD meta-analyses, data-sharing platforms are meant to supplement—not replace—working directly with original researchers to obtain clinical trial IPD. Platforms can allow IPD meta-analysts to find studies and also benefit from independent review of proposals. Waldstreicher's company and others will work with researchers to try to provide data for analyses that cannot be completed within the platform or within the company's secure website. Roberts agreed that her company and others do try to meet the needs of data requesters when the data of interest are housed in multiple platforms. She said these efforts are currently case by case, but also said that she was hopeful for a broader solution in the future.

Baigent shared his experience with seeking datasets from 19 placebo-controlled trials conducted by different statin manufacturers. He said he had experienced manufacturer reluctance in providing the data directly, and was instructed to go through the data-sharing platforms that each company was using. Multiple problems were encountered, he said (e.g., delays in obtaining permission to extract data, inability to upload software efficiently). The solution, he said, was to directly lobby within the companies to seek access to the IPD, and, in many cases, agreements were ultimately reached. Baigent shared his understanding that companies have a vested interest in using their own platforms that they have been developing, but he added that there are also circumstances when it should be understood from the start that certain data would need to be maintained locally by the researchers. Even when an analyst is interested in datasets from only one company or platform, Baigent noted, the inability to house data locally means that meta-analysts must upload their own analysis software behind the platform firewall.

Mandating Data Sharing

Tim Feeney asked whether ICMJE might have a role to play in promoting the cultural shift toward data sharing through establishing publication requirements, as was done for prospective trial registration. Humphreys said that, at a recent meeting of the Science and Technology Select Committee of the UK Parliament, an ICMJE journal editor suggested that idea. She said the editor believed that ICMJE could require that study results be posted in a registry prior to publication. Humphreys added that the same concept could apply to funders. She said a cross-funder survey of 174 clinical researchers found that half believed funders should mandate sharing of funded data, and half believed that mandating data would lead to sharing of data that are not meaningful, simply to meet the requirement. Concerns were also expressed that it is too early to mandate sharing data because there is no system yet to award credit for sharing.

Baigent summarized that there is broad agreement that data from randomized controlled clinical trials should be shared. The pooled clinical trial data supporting an IPD meta-analysis, however, is often not suitable for sharing, as the data sharing agreement (DSA) with each one of the multiple trial sponsors usually requires a confidentiality agreement for the data user to be allowed to maintain the data locally within their institution. IPD meta-analysts are often criticized for not sharing the data supporting the analysis, he said, but it is often forgotten that they do not own data from individual trials, and are generally legally prohibited from sharing with third parties due to data-sharing agreements. He urged caution in creating rules that would potentially place these high-value projects in legal jeopardy.

Roberts agreed and recalled the remarks made about the definition of "all trials." There are other reasons why sharing data might not be possible or meaningful. Nurnberger agreed with the need for caution regarding mandates. She suggested that the potential sharing of derived datasets could be discussed when negotiating the DSA, including how to ensure traceability of the data.

Datasets from Tertiary Analyses

Alex Sherman raised the special issue of sharing information from tertiary analyses. When shared data or biospecimens (e.g., cerebrospinal fluid, DNA) are used for omics and generate large sequencing data files, should these omics data files be associated with the shared original data? Or are these sequence files the property of the researcher who did the sequencing?

Humphreys and Roberts were not aware of any agreed standard on this issue. In general, Humphreys said, journals require that the source of any data used is acknowledged in the publication (e.g., persistent identifier for the dataset used), and Vivli will store the derived datasets. Humphreys suggested that if an IRP was used for access to the primary datasets, and then the same IRP is used for access to the derived dataset, it would reduce the need to reach out to the multiple primary data generators every time there was interest in using the derived dataset. Nurnberger said each of the original datasets used to create the derived dataset will likely have licensing or sharing agreements that indicate the sharing expectations for the derived dataset. In addition, for the scholarly record, it is important to share the derived dataset in some way, and she advocated for the use of dynamic data citations to the original datasets. Roberts suggested that further discussion was needed between data originators and researchers on this topic.

Specialists in Data Sharing

Matthew Sydes recalled that the remarks about research team members focused on data sharing and about engaging the data management experts in library services. He asked whether organizations conducting clinical trials should be establishing positions for specialists in data sharing. Roberts said that in her company of about 7,500 employees, several staff members specialize in data sharing. The best solution for an organization depends on its size, structure, and other factors, she said. A question to be addressed, Humphreys said, is how those positions would be funded and sustained. Humphreys then shared support for the concept of a central core resource of dedicated experts, rather than a person on each trial team being assigned the task for a given project. As an example, she said that a pilot being conducted in Ireland uses a portion of the funding from each grant to cover the cost of 15 data stewards in different institutions across Ireland, with each project also contributing a small portion of their total budget.[15] Nurnberger agreed with the concept

[15] See https://www.hrb.ie/news/latest-news/news-story/article/hrb-to-offer-training-opportunity-to-create-irelands-first-fair-data-stewards (accessed March 15, 2020) for more information on the pilot program.

of trial teams having access to a core, centralized service of specialists in data management and sharing. Baigent said his department of about 600 staff members is establishing a team that will be responsible for data sharing. Large departments generate volumes of data, and there is a need for data-sharing expertise that is maintained by institutions, he noted. Humphreys added that data stewards have a role up-front in the development of data management plans or output management plans. These data stewards, she said, can provide perspectives on what the costs of data sharing might be for a given project—which can then be included in a funding application.

Pathways to Sharing: Precompetitive Consortia, Direct Collaboration, and Platforms

Ida Sim summarized the three main models of sharing data that have been discussed throughout the workshop, noting that each has different requirements and provides different support to researchers: (1) the precompetitive consortium model that brings groups of investigators together to pool data to discuss a research question (e.g., WWARN); (2) direct collaboration between data generators and data users for reanalysis of the data; and (3) facilitation of sharing by an independent third-party (i.e., platform). Sim observed that the platform model has the highest resource requirements for preparing data for sharing and processing requests for access. The task now is to reflect on where and how to provide enabling support to return the most value.

Humphreys added that the models must be FAIR and transparent. She suggested that some researchers are left out of the data sharing that takes place through consortia and direct contact (i.e., the data are not accessible to them by those pathways). Baigent said there is value to collaborating directly with those who have the greatest knowledge of the data and who can help interpret the overall results. Collaboration and collective interpretation by researchers with very different perspectives can also lead to better science, he said.

Nurnberger proposed a fourth model, in which clinical trial data are used by others outside of the clinical trial community, in particular, for machine learning or applications of artificial intelligence. Some important questions to consider going forward, Nurnberger pointed out, include Where will research go next? What needs to be done so that data are useful 10 years from now? How can the investments made in these studies be extended even further?

CLOSING REMARKS: FINDING VALUE AS WE MOVE FORWARD

Waldstreicher reflected on the progress made since the 2015 Institute of Medicine report *Sharing Clinical Trial Data: Maximizing Benefits, Minimizing Risk* (IOM, 2015). She observed that this workshop included discussions about sharing data across platforms for meta-analyses—while 5 years ago, the discussion was simply about how to facilitate data sharing, and the platforms of today did not exist.

Waldstreicher also pointed out some limitations of frequently used metrics, noting the insufficiency of measuring success by simply counting the number of publications resulting from data sharing. Other secondary uses of data that should be measured were discussed, including the use of data to inform methods development or to improve the statistical power of new studies. The importance of learning from failure was also raised; sharing data from failed studies is important, she said, so that researchers across companies and sectors can work together. Waldstreicher reiterated the point by Deborah Zarin that the possibility of auditing trials could help "raise the bar" and inspire researchers to collect data in a fashion that better facilitates sharing.

During the past 5 years that data sharing has been increasing, none of the anticipated unintended consequences have materialized, Waldstreicher noted. Across all of the platforms discussed and stakeholder perspectives shared, there were, for example, no reports of attempts to reidentify participants, no purported safety issues, and no principal investigators who had their findings "scooped" by others analyzing data they had shared.

Work still needs to be done, Waldstreicher said. There was much discussion about the need to enable analysis of data across trials and across platforms, and there was discussion of the merits of having a single platform. Each stakeholder generates data for their own purposes. Companies need data for product licensure, Waldstreicher added, while for researchers in academia data can be a currency for career advancement. Ultimately though, data are generated for the public good, "to make a difference for patients," she said. The perspectives shared by Moses Taylor, Jr., and Sharon Terry, Waldstreicher noted, illustrate the importance of secondary use of data both for general public health and for individual participants—as well as the need to keep the participant perspective at the core of data sharing. She reiterated a phrase that Bernard Lo had coined saying that "data sharing is important because this is the science that is the foundation of medicine and medical care."

Drazen agreed with Waldstreicher that there has been encouraging progress over the past few years, and the question now is how best to move forward. He suggested stratifying the different types of clinical trials that are conducted based on the relative level of interest in the data generated. First, there are trials that are designed to inform and influence clinical practice. Often, these trials are sponsored by companies developing products, but they may also be sponsored by agencies such as the National Institutes of Health in the United States and MRC in the United Kingdom. Designed for regulatory submission, these trials are well documented and conform to principles of good data husbandry. He pointed out that numerous decisions can be made over the course of a study, so there should be a focus on improving habits so this information is documented in a way that makes it easy to understand how the study was conducted.

The second type of trial analyzes the effect of an intervention to better understand the biology of disease. Drazen said this type of trial is generally smaller (i.e., less statistical power), and there may be less interest in these datasets. However, the data may be of interest to researchers seeking to better understand disease biology, so "good enough" data husbandry is still important.

Finally, numerous trials are carried out to examine biological or physiological endpoints. Data from these types of studies are potentially shareable and therefore should involve some consideration of what would be minimally sufficient for data sharing.

Drazen then outlined a few general categories of data use. One category includes cases in which data are used either to check the outcome of a trial or to combine data across trials for advancing medical knowledge and practice. While these types of data applications can be of value to the medical and academic communities, there are concerns to be considered. Drazen observed that 5 years ago, trialists were concerned about potential adversarial uses of their data. Today, adversarial thinking on the part of trialists has evolved to be more flexible and focus on the potential advantages of data sharing. He added that third party platforms can serve as valuable intermediaries in this process. Another category of data use described by Drazen includes cases in which data are used to supplement a trial that lacks statistical power to address a particular question. Collaborative approaches to combine data from across multiple studies can help to advance the field, Drazen said. He noted that researchers seem willing to engage in this type of collaborative work, and he hopes to see more of this in the future. An additional category of data use, Drazen added, includes the application of shared data to examine the result of placebo treatment for people with a particular condition. This application might use shared data to help power a trial (e.g., to determine the frequency of a given complication when no treatment is administered).

These types of trials and categories of use can come together in many ways, Drazen said. In moving forward, he suggested that mandates for sharing may not be needed. Funders can be influential in promoting sharing. Drazen suggested they might require data sharing for large-scale clinical trials, while encouraging data sharing for trials to understand the biology of a disease. Underlying all types of trials, Drazen reiterated, is the need to adopt standards that better facilitate the sharing and use of datasets. He stated that by keeping the focus on patients and improving care, everything else will fall into place.

Appendix A

References

ART (Anturane Reinfarction Trial) Research Group. 1980. Sulfinpyrazone in the prevention of sudden death after myocardial infarction. *New England Journal of Medicine* 302(5):250–256.

Baggerly, K. A., and K. R. Coombes. 2009. Deriving chemosensitivity from cell lines: Forensic bioinformatics and reproducible research in high-throughput biology. *Annals of Applied Statistics* 3(4):1309–1334.

Baron, J. A., R. S. Sandler, R. S. Bresalier, A. Lanas, D. G. Morton, R. Riddell, E. R. Iverson, and D. L. Demets. 2008. Cardiovascular events associated with rofecoxib: Final analysis of the APPROVe trial. *Lancet* 372(9651):1756–1764.

Bertagnolli, M. M., O. Sartor, B. A. Chabner, M. L. Rothenberg, S. Khozin, C. Hugh-Jones, D. M. Reese, and M. J. Murphy. 2017. Advantages of a truly open-access data-sharing model. *New England Journal of Medicine* 376(12):1178–1181.

Bresalier, R. S., R. S. Sandler, H. Quan, J. A. Bolognese, B. Oxenius, K. Horgan, C. Lines, R. Riddell, D. Morton, A. Lanas, M. A. Konstam, J. A. Baron, and the Adenomatous Polyp Prevention on Vioxx (APPROVe) Trial Investigators. 2005. Cardiovascular events associated with rofecoxib in a colorectal adenoma chemoprevention trial. *New England Journal of Medicine* 352(11):1092–1102.

Bristow, M. R., L. A. Saxon, J. Boehmer, S. Krueger, D. A. Kass, T. De Marco, P. Carson, L. DiCarlo, D. DeMets, B. G. White, D. W. DeVries, A. M. Feldman, and Comparison of Medical Therapy, Pacing, and Defibrillation in Heart Failure (COMPANION) Investigators. 2004. Cardiac resynchronization therapy with or without an implantable defibrillator in advanced chronic heart failure. *New England Journal of Medicine* 350:2140–2150.

Corbett, M., F. Chehadah, M. Biswas, T. Moe-Byrne, S. Palmer, M. Soares, M. Walton, M. Harden, P. Ho, N. Woolacott, and L. Bojke. 2017. Certolizumab pegol and secukinumab for treating active psoriatic arthritis following inadequate response to disease-modifying antirheumatic drugs: A systematic review and economic evaluation. *Health Technology Assessment* 21(56):1–326.

Duma, N., J. Vera Aguilera, J. Paludo, C. L. Haddox, M. Gonzalez Velez, Y. Wang, K. Leventakos, J. M. Hubbard, A. S. Mansfield, R. S. Go, and A. A. Adjei. 2018. Representation of minorities and women in oncology clinical trials: Review of the past 14 years. *Journal of Oncology Practice* 14(1):e1–e10.

Gamble, C., A. Krishan, D. Stocken, S. Lewis, E. Juszczak, C. Doré, P. R. Williamson, D. G. Altman, A. Montgomery, P. Lim, J. Berlin, S. Senn, S. Day, Y. Barbachano, and E. Loder. 2017. Guidelines for the content of statistical analysis plans in clinical trials. *JAMA* 318(23):2337–2343.

Gay, H. C., A. S. Baldridge, and M. D. Huffman. 2017. Feasibility, process, and outcomes of cardiovascular clinical trial data sharing: A reproduction analysis of the SMART-AF Trial. *JAMA Cardiology* 2(12):1375–1379.

Gritz, E. R., C. Dresler, and L. Sarna. 2005. Smoking, the missing drug interaction in clinical trials: Ignoring the obvious. *Cancer Epidemiology, Biomarkers & Prevention* 14(10):2287–2293.

IOM (Institute of Medicine). 2012a. *Envisioning a transformed clinical trials enterprise in the United States: Establishing an agenda for 2020: Workshop summary*. Washington, DC: The National Academies Press.

IOM. 2012b. *Evolution of translational omics: Lessons learned and the path forward*. Washington, DC: The National Academies Press.

IOM. 2013. *Sharing clinical research data: Workshop summary*. Washington, DC: The National Academies Press.

IOM. 2015. *Sharing clinical trial data: Maximizing benefits, minimizing risk*. Washington, DC: The National Academies Press.

Kochhar, S., B. Knoppers, C. Gamble, A. Chant, J. Koplan, and G. S. Humphreys. 2019. Clinical trial data sharing: Here's the challenge. *BMJ Open* 9(8):e032334.

Kratz, J. E., and C. Strasser. 2015. Researcher perspectives on publication and peer review of data. *PLOS ONE* 10(2):e0117619.

Kush, R. D. 2014. What the patient should order. *Science Translational Medicine* 1(3):3cm3.

Kush, R., and M. Goldman. 2014. Fostering responsible data sharing through standards. *New England Journal of Medicine* 370(23):2163–2165.

Land, S. R., B. A. Toll, C. M. Moinpour, S. A. Mitchell, J. S. Ostroff, D. K. Hatsukami, S. A. Duffy, E. R. Gritz, N. A. Rigotti, T. H. Brandon, S. A. Prindiville, L. P. Sarna, R. A. Schnoll, R. S. Herbst, P. M. Cinciripini, S. J. Leischow, C. M. Dresler, M. C. Fiore, and G. W. Warren. 2016. Research priorities, measures, and recommendations for assessment of tobacco use in clinical cancer research. *Clinical Cancer Research* 22(8):1907–1913.

Lo, B., and D. J. DeMets. 2016. Incentives for clinical trialists to share data. *New England Journal of Medicine* 375(12):1112–1115.

Mbuagbaw, L., L. Guglielmetti, C. Hewison, N. Bakare, M. Bastard, E. Caumes, M. Fréchet-Jachym, J. Robert, N. Veziris, N. Khachatryan, T. Kotrikadze, A. Hayrapetyan, Z. Avaliani, H. J. Schünemann, and C. Lienhardt. 2019. Outcomes of bedaquiline treatment in patients with multidrug-resistant tuberculosis. *Emerging Infectious Diseases* 25(5):936–943.

Mello, M. M., V. Lieou, and S. N. Goodman. 2018. Clinical trial participants' views of the risks and benefits of data sharing. *New England Journal of Medicine* 378(23):2202–2211.

Ohmann, C., R. Banzi, S. Canham, S. Battaglia, M. Matei, C. Ariyo, L. Becnel, B. Bierer, S. Bowers, L. Clivio, M. Dias, C. Druml, H. Faure, M. Fenner, J. Galvez, D. Ghersi, C. Gluud, T. Groves, P. Houston, G. Karam, D. Kalra, R. L. Knowles, K. Krleža-Jerić, C. Kubiak, W. Kuchinke, R. Kush, A. Lukkarinen, P. S. Marques, A. Newbigging, J. O'Callaghan, P. Ravaud, I. Schlünder, D. Shanahan, H. Sitter, D. Spalding, C. Tudur Smith, P. van Reusel, E. van Veen, G. R. Visser, J. Wilson, and J. Demotes-Mainard. 2017. Sharing and reuse of individual participant data from clinical trials: Principles and recommendations. *BMJ Open* 7(12):e018647.

Peters, E. N., E. Torres, B. A. Toll, K. M. Cummings, E. R. Gritz, A. Hyland, R. S. Herbst, J. R. Marshall, and W. G. Warren. 2012. Tobacco assessment in actively accruing National Cancer Institute Cooperative Group Program Clinical Trials. *Journal of Clinical Oncology* 30(23):2869–2875.

Regnante, J. M., N. A. Richie, L. Fashoyin-Aje, M. Vichnin, M. Ford, U. B. Roy, K. Turner, L. L. Hall, E. Gonzalez, N. Esnaola, L. T. Clark, H. C. Adams 3rd, O. B. Alese, K. Gogineni, L. McNeill, D. Petereit, I. Sargeant, J. Dang, C. Obasaju, Q. Highsmith, S. C. Lee, S. C. Hoover, E. L. Williams, and M. S. Chen, Jr. 2019. U.S. cancer centers of excellence strategies for increased inclusion of racial and ethnic minorities in clinical trials. *Journal of Oncology Practice* 15(4):e289–e299.

Ross, J. S., J. Waldstreicher, S. Bamford, J. A. Berlin, K. Childers, N. R. Desai, G. Gamble, C. P. Gross, R. Kuntz, R. Lehman, P. Lins, S. A. Morris, J. D. Ritchie, and H. M. Krumholz. 2018. Overview and experience of the YODA Project with clinical trial data sharing after 5 years. *Scientific Data* 5:180268.

Solomon, S. D., J. J. McMurray, M. A. Pfeffer, J. Wittes, R. Fowler, P. Finn, W. F. Anderson, A. Zauber, E. Hawk, M. Bertagnolli, and the Adenoma Prevention with Celecoxib (APC) Study Investigators. 2005. Cardiovascular risk associated with celecoxib in a clinical trial for colorectal adenoma prevention. *New England Journal of Medicine* 352(11):1071–1080.

Solomon, S. D., J. Wittes, P. V. Finn, R. Fowler, J. Viner, M. M. Bertagnolli, N. Arber, B. Levin, C. L. Meinert, B. Martin, J. L. Pater, P. E. Goss, P. Lance, S. Obara, E. Y. Chew, J. Kim, G. Arndt, E. Hawk, and the Cross Trial Safety Assessment Group. 2008. Cardiovascular risk of celecoxib in 6 randomized placebo-controlled trials: The Cross Trial safety analysis. *Circulation* 117(16):2104–2113.

SPRINT (Systolic Blood Pressure Intervention Trial) Research Group, J. T. Wright Jr., J. D. Williamson, P. K. Whelton, J. K. Snyder, K. M. Sink, M. V. Rocco, D. M. Reboussin, M. Rahman, S. Oparil, C. E. Lewis, P. L. Kimmel, K. C. Johnson, D. C. Goff, Jr., L. J. Fine, J. A. Cutler, W. C. Cushman, A. K. Cheung, and W. T. Ambrosius. 2015. A randomized trial of intensive versus standard blood-pressure control. *New England Journal of Medicine* 373(22):2103–2116.

Sydes, M. R., and D. Ashby. 2017. Data authorship as an incentive to data sharing. *New England Journal of Medicine* 377(4):402.

Temple, R., and G. W. Pledger. 1980. The FDA's critique of the Anturane Reinfarction Trial. *New England Journal of Medicine* 303(25):1488–1492.

Tudur Smith, C., S. Nevitt, D. Appelbe, R. Appleton, P. Dixon, J. Harrison, A. Marson, P. Williamson, and E. Tremain. 2017. Resource implications of preparing individual participant data from a clinical trial to share with external researchers. *Trials* 18(1):319.

van Den Eynden, V. G. Knight, A. Vlad, B. Radler, C. Tenopir, D. Leon, F. Manista, J. Whitworth, and L. Corti. 2016. *Survey of Wellcome researchers and their attitudes to open research. Technical Report*. https://researchonline.lshtm.ac.uk/id/eprint/3332696/1/TowardsOpenResearch.pdf (accessed February 10, 2020).

Varnai, P., M. C. Rentel., P. Simmonds., T. A. Sharp, B. Mostert, and T. de Jongh. 2014. *Assessing the research potential of access to clinical trial data. A report to the Wellcome Trust*. Technopolis Group (UK). https://wellcome.ac.uk/sites/default/files/assessing-research-potential-of-access-to-clinical-trials-data-wellcome-mar15.pdf (accessed February 10, 2020).

Zarin, D. A., and T. Tse. 2016. Sharing individual participant data (IPD) within the context of the trial reporting system (TRS). *PLOS Medicine* 13(1):e1001946.

Appendix B

Workshop Agenda

Sharing Clinical Trial Data: Challenges and a Way Forward:
A Workshop

November 18–19, 2019
National Academy of Sciences Building, Great Hall
2101 Constitution Avenue, NW, Washington, DC 20418

WORKSHOP OBJECTIVES

Following release of the 2015 Institute of Medicine report *Sharing Clinical Trial Data: Maximizing Benefits, Minimizing Risks*:

- Consider the value and potential risks/costs of sharing clinical trial data for key stakeholders, including clinical trialists, sponsors, primary and secondary researchers, and patients;
- Review the current landscape of clinical trial data sharing and reuse across public and private sectors (e.g., policies, platforms, collaborations, data sharing culture, published research output);

- Examine use cases and trends from across public and private sectors when it comes to success, failure, lessons learned, and value;
- Consider the perspectives and expectations of primary and secondary researchers, clinical trial participants, patient organizations, research sponsors (pharmaceutical companies and nonprofit organizations), journals, institutions, and federal agencies; and
- Discuss next step opportunities for stakeholders to better harmonize incentives, policy, data standards, and governance to encourage the sharing and reuse of clinical trial data.

DAY 1: November 18, 2019

8:00 a.m. **Breakfast available in the Great Hall**

8:30 a.m. **Welcome and opening remarks**

Jeffrey M. Drazen, *Workshop Co-Chair*
Group Editor
New England Journal of Medicine

Joanne Waldstreicher, *Workshop Co-Chair*
Chief Medical Officer
Johnson & Johnson

Session I: The Current Landscape of Clinical Trial Data Sharing and Reuse

Session Objectives:

- Consider the value and potential risks/costs of sharing clinical trial data for key stakeholders, including clinical trialists, sponsors, primary and secondary researchers, and patients
- Review the current landscape of clinical trial data sharing and reuse across public and private sectors (e.g., policies, platforms, collaborations, data sharing culture)
- Examine case studies and trends from across public and private sectors when it comes to success, failure, lessons learned, and value

9:00 a.m. **Landscape overview by session moderators**

BERNARD LO
President and Chief Executive Officer
The Greenwall Foundation

DEBORAH ZARIN
Director
Program for the Advancement of the Clinical Trials Enterprise
Multi-Regional Clinical Trials Center
Brigham and Women's Hospital and Harvard

9:20 a.m. **Policies in practice: Lessons learned**

A researcher perspective
HARLAN KRUMHOLZ
Harold H. Hines Jr. Professor of Medicine
Yale School of Medicine

A funder perspective
LYRIC JORGENSON
Deputy Director
Office of Science Policy
National Institutes of Health

An independent review panel perspective
SONALI KOCHHAR
Medical Director
Global Healthcare Consulting

A patient perspective
MOSES TAYLOR, JR.
Participant
SPRINT Trial

10:20 a.m. **Data sharing platforms: Use cases**

Vivli
REBECCA LI
Executive Director
Vivli

The YODA Project
JOSEPH ROSS
Professor of Medicine and Public Health
Yale School of Medicine

SOAR
FRANK ROCKHOLD
Professor of Biostatistics and Bioinformatics
Duke University Medical Center

ClinicalStudyDataRequest.com
SCOTT SHAUNESSY
Chair
ClinicalStudyDataRequest.com

11:20 a.m. **BREAK**

11:50 a.m. **Panel discussion: Striking a balance between benefit/value and risk/cost—is the juice worth the squeeze?**

A data analyst perspective
DAVID DEMETS
Professor Emeritus
Department of Biostatistics and Medical Informatics
University of Wisconsin–Madison

A publisher perspective
JEFFREY M. DRAZEN
Group Editor
New England Journal of Medicine

A patient perspective
DEBORAH C. PEEL
Founder and President
Patient Privacy Rights

12:35 p.m. ***Moderated audience discussion with the panel***

1:00 p.m. **BREAK** (Lunch available in the Great Hall)

Session II: Key Challenges in Clinical Trial Data Sharing and Reuse

Session Objectives:

- Discuss key challenges to clinical trial data sharing and reuse by including use cases
- Consider the perspectives and expectations of clinical trial participants, patients, research sponsors (pharmaceutical companies and nonprofit organizations), journals, academic researchers and institutions, institutional review boards, and federal agencies

1:30 p.m. **Opening remarks by session moderators**

TIMOTHY COETZEE
Chief Advocacy, Services, and Research Officer
National Multiple Sclerosis Society

DINA PALTOO
Assistant Director
Policy Development
National Library of Medicine
National Institutes of Health

1:45 p.m. **Panel discussion: Data interoperability and platform usability**

Use case: Population data
ERNEST HAWK
Vice President and Division Head
Cancer Prevention and Population Sciences
MD Anderson

Use case: Meta-analysis
TIANJING LI
Associate Professor
University of Colorado Denver

A platform perspective
BILL LOUV
President
Project Data Sphere

2:15 p.m. ***Moderated audience discussion with the panel***

2:45 p.m. **Panel discussion: Infrastructure sustainability**

A funder perspective
GEORGINA HUMPHREYS
Clinical Data Sharing Manager
Wellcome Trust

A business perspective
PANDURANG KULKARNI
Chief Analytics Officer R&D
Vice President
Biometrics and Advanced Analytics
Eli Lilly and Company

A platform perspective
SEAN COADY
Program Officer
National Heart, Lung, and Blood Institute
National Institutes of Health

3:15 p.m. ***Moderated audience discussion with the panel***

3:45 p.m. **BREAK**

4:15 p.m. **Panel discussion: Challenges and disincentives for sharing and using data**

Use case: Statistical replication

A researcher perspective
MATTHEW SYDES
Professor of Clinical Trials and Methodology
Medical Research Council Clinical Trials Unit
University College London

A sponsor perspective
RAMIN DARON
Vice President, Data Architecture and Technology
Takeda Pharmaceuticals

A patient perspective
SHARON TERRY
President and Chief Executive Officer
Genetic Alliance

4:45 p.m. ***Moderated audience discussion with the panel***

Day 1 Reflections

5:15 p.m. **Finding value as we move forward**

Jeffrey M. Drazen, *Workshop Co-Chair*
Group Editor
New England Journal of Medicine

Joanne Waldstreicher, *Workshop Co-Chair*
Chief Medical Officer
Johnson & Johnson

5:30 p.m. **ADJOURN WORKSHOP DAY 1**

DAY 2: November 19, 2019

8:00 a.m. **Breakfast available in the Great Hall**

8:30 a.m. **Welcome and overview of Day 1**

Jeffrey M. Drazen, *Workshop Co-Chair*
Group Editor
New England Journal of Medicine

Joanne Waldstreicher, *Workshop Co-Chair*
Chief Medical Officer
Johnson & Johnson

Session III: Finding Value in Sharing Clinical Trial Data

Session Objectives:

- Discuss next step opportunities for stakeholders to better align incentives, and implement policy, technology, and governance that encourage the sharing and reuse of clinical trial data:
  - Explore opportunities for overcoming technical barriers
  - Explore opportunities for addressing cultural barriers
  - Discuss possible solutions/next steps going forward

8:45 a.m. **Panel discussion: Overcoming usability and sustainability challenges**

Moderator
IDA SIM
Professor of Medicine
University of California, San Francisco, School of Medicine

A data user perspective
MARK HELFAND
Professor of Medicine, Medical Informatics, and Clinical Epidemiology
Oregon Health & Science University

A data generator/sharer perspective
MONICA BERTAGNOLLI
Professor of Surgery
Harvard Medical School

A platform perspective
REBECCA KUSH
Chief Scientific Officer
Elligo Health Research

9:30 a.m. *Moderated audience discussion with the panel*

10:00 a.m. **BREAK**

10:30 a.m. **Panel discussion: Looking forward: Incentivizing data sharing and reuse**

Moderator and sponsor perspective
LIZ ROBERTS
Senior Director and Global Public Policy Lead
UCB Biosciences

A researcher perspective
COLIN BAIGENT
Deputy Director
Clinical Trial Service Unit and Epidemiological Studies Unit
Oxford University

An institutional perspective
AMY NURNBERGER
Program Head
Data Management Services
Massachusetts Institute of Technology

A funder perspective
GEORGINA HUMPHREYS
Clinical Data Sharing Manager
Wellcome Trust

11:45 a.m. ***Moderated audience discussion with the panel***

12:15 p.m. **Next Steps**

JEFFREY M. DRAZEN, *Workshop Co-Chair*
Group Editor
New England Journal of Medicine

JOANNE WALDSTREICHER, *Workshop Co-Chair*
Chief Medical Officer
Johnson & Johnson

12:30 p.m. **ADJOURN WORKSHOP DAY 2**